LET'S LIGHTEN UP

Replenish What Makes Us Strong
*
Enjoy The Very Best of Health
*
Always Catch The Rain

By Pete Egoscue, Author of **PAIN FREE**
with Roger Gittines

Egoscue Method Books / San Diego

LET'S LIGHTEN UP

An Egoscue Method Book/March 2010

All rights reserved.

Copyright © 2010 Pete Egoscue.

Photos (instructional) Copyright © The Egoscue Method.

Dust Jacket Cover Photo and other Art and Icon Photos by License from Big Stock Photo.

Book and Cover Design by DataStream Content Solutions, LLC.

Copy Editing by MyCopyEditor.com.

Index by Twin Oaks Indexing.

Library of Congress control number: 2010920783
Egoscue, Pete, 1945–
Let's lighten up: replenish what makes us strong, enjoy the very best of health, always catch the rain / by Pete Egoscue, with Roger Gittines.

p.   cm.

ISBN 978-0-615-34124-8

Health–Exercise therapy.   I. Gittines, Roger.   II. Title.

My book is dedicated to the wonder and mystery of the human mind, body and spirit that reveals itself through the crystal lens of peace of mind.

Acknowledgments

Most authors tend to avoid tipping off their readers to the importance of various themes and topics. The reticence is probably nothing more than common-sense civility since it may seem presumptuous and discourteous to suggest that readers can't make up their own minds without prompting from higher authority. Okay, I'll start with a denial. I am not writing this with intent to prompt. What I am up to is—gasp!—truth-telling. Awareness is without doubt my primary theme in the pages you are about to encounter. There are many gateways to awareness; some I don't even know about yet. But it is appropriate that the first one that I come to here is gratitude.

By writing and publishing a book an author puts himself in debt to hundreds of people, including his readers. Awareness entered through the portal of gratitude is at first a shock. There is a whiff of lost independence, inadequacy and false humility. But it quickly gives way to the realization that if I did not need help, I'd be better off in the business of carving stone tablets, not writing books. Being in need of help and being helped are no sins. Public declaration of the debt, no matter how inadequate the act of expression, and the genuine gratitude it represents are powerful means of redemption. Thanks to your help I've been able to do my best to help others. For that—and for this construction of ink, ideas, paper, passion and glue—I am deeply grateful.

"Nothing can bring you peace but yourself."

– Ralph Waldo Emerson

You Know: An Informal Introduction

This book is a celebration. It is about the whole world—your world, your life.

About beliefs, actions and consequences; about the truth concerning your deepest thoughts, where they come from and what effect they have on your health and well-being.

Both mutable facts of constant change and immutable perceptions born of change fascinate me. Our home planet, a shimmering blue-and-green orb first seen in Apollo Mission photos barely forty years ago, is already a much different place. Five centuries after Columbus boldly sailed west to reach the East, the fundamental rounded and rounding shape of things seems to have been flattened by technology and relentless systemic upheaval (at least, that is, if you believe the best-selling books and popular newspaper columns of Thomas Friedman and other likeminded commentators). Science has been busy producing one dramatic breakthrough after another. Yet why are we so sick? In so much pain? So fearful? What's going on? Why are we all searching outside of ourselves—in pill bottles, cups super-sized like buckets brimming with enough high-fructose corn syrup to caramelize your pancreas with one sip, oceans of caffeine and booming, empty stimulation via the blipping, beeping gadgetry of the newest new 'normal'–scratching for just enough energy to survive the day?

The answer is hidden in the labyrinth of unintended consequences cut through the crust of reality itself by modern scientific methodology, by its profound impact on commerce, medical training, values and the treatment of human pain and suffering. As you trudge along the narrow passageway of that confusing maze, I invite you to imagine with me that just around the next blind corner on a wall inscribed in gold lettering is an observation, inspired by spiritual teachings, known as the Noble Eightfold Path of Buddhism: "Pain is inevitable; suffering is optional."

Who left the message? A seeker–someone just like you.

Pain causes devastating physical and spiritual suffering when we erroneously conclude that there is no choice: Any relief or release is ultimately chimerical and comes at a great price–immobility, lost dignity and the sacrifice of personal strength, independence and security. Burdened by pessimism, we despair that our bodies are too complicated and fragile for us to understand what causes pain, much less do anything about it and regain full health.

Unlike my previous books–pages of factoids supporting what I believe about chronic musculoskeletal system pain–I intend to remind you of what you already know: All truth dwells within; only awareness provides access to the enlightenment of ancient wisdom forged from experience. This book is about renewing that awareness, about how to know the inner truth about your health. Humankind possesses roughly a million years of practical, operational experience in dealing with pain. Yet starting comparatively recently, many of us have been beguiled by the notion that medical science knows so much about the inner workings of the body that this or that drug or surgical procedure–often with damaging side effects–offer the only real hope to those who are in pain.

Sounds reasonable. But fortunately when we try to tell our bodies to shut up, butt out and get on with whatever program that is being presented to us by caring, dedicated, highly intelligent, and awesomely well-educated men and women, a million years' worth of actually knowing better–knowing ourselves more thoroughly than any other human being could possibly manage–kicks in. Indeed, we may not act wisely on that knowledge, yet ignorance is a poor excuse for that particular form of bliss. We know: Seeking to know is what we strive so long and hard to do. Confronted by the experts our emotions, driven by our hyper-vigilant sensory perceptions, refuse to surrender a deep set of beliefs forged from urgent watch fires of experience that still remain hot to the touch. This is a book of absolute optimism rooted in an amazing, bullet-proof, nearly perfect belief system that functions in harmony with an equally amazing cellular/molecular-level command-and-control juggernaut.

Juggernaut? Is that the correct noun? Probably not. But a vocabulary capable of describing a mechanism that directs 60 trillion cells in a whirling, lifelong dance of unimaginable precision and complexity is still being assembled. In this case, the inaptly named juggernaut, partnered with the almost too familiar, too trite rubric of spiritual belief, is actually relying on stubborn disbelief (or, at the very least, obstinate doubt) to keep us skeptical and alive long enough to rediscover the healing power of inner truth.

Bravo! That's the good news. For a change there is no bad news.

Wallow in optimism. Have fun with the pages that follow, since having fun is usually a sign we are doing the right thing. Then go for it–make a choice. Find lasting enjoyment; in every sense be *en joyed*.

En riched.

Remember—and rejoice that the memory persists within— suffering is optional. You have the power to choose between sickness and health, hope and fear. Truth is a feeling, not a fact. Feel your way to the best of health.

Pete Egoscue

Contents

About disclaimers, deciders, and decisions

I believe this book validates the wisdom, knowledge and experience you have about your own health. Because you know more about it than anyone else, I offer the following heart-felt counsel. It's always a good idea to seek out and carefully listen to intelligent and perceptive health care advice. It's always a bad idea to act on that advice, including my own, without fully accepting your paramount role in safeguarding the perfect health that comes to us all as a precious human birthright and legacy.

Pete

Illustrations

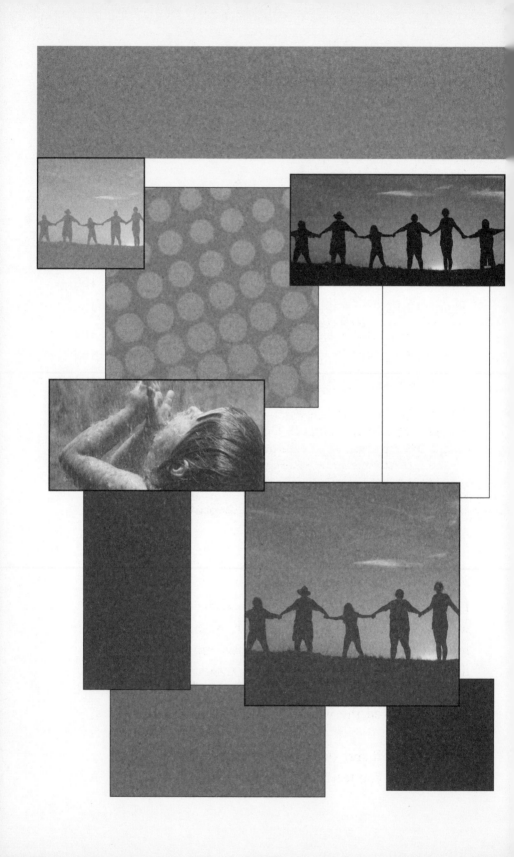

Good Cause

"People say that what we're seeking is a meaning for life. I don't think that's what we're really seeking.... [W]hat we're seeking is an experience of being alive, so ... that we have resonances within our innermost being and reality [and] ... actually feel the rapture of being alive."

—Joseph Campbell

I know a guy who for thirty years—in the course of writing four books, taking part in more than a half-million clinical consultations, speaking at hundreds of seminars, giving media interviews, and conducting health workshops and classroom discussions—asked the wrong question over and over again.

Yeah, but it sure did sound right:

"How do you feel?"

See what I mean? What could possibly be wrong about that? A lot. Now we know there was a trapdoor built into the sentence, hidden between the "do" and the "you." When the question was asked, the floor suddenly, silently, dropped away and most of those who were trying their best to answer vanished.

Actually that's a slight overstatement. They did not vanish–a meaningful answer disappeared.

A fine, serviceable question–*How do you feel?* It seems to cover a lot of ground and leave enough space for "I feel cold," "I feel thirsty," "... feel good ...," "... bad ...," "... better ...," or "... worse...." A quick inventory of what's most bothersome. Even so, in practice, there is only spare headroom for pain, if there is actually pain in the neighborhood or if there is a fresh memory of a recent visitation. And if people happen to be pain-free when the question is asked, most tend to cautiously double-check in case pain has slipped by them unnoticed, and most other feelings–particularly those that can be transitory and fragile, like happiness and peace of mind–are often overlooked.

Here's a more-or-less accurate translation of "How do you feel?": What's really being asked is–"Do you feel pain? Where? Does it hurt more or less or not at all when you ...?" (Fill in the blank with one of a thousand reasonably sound diagnostic techniques.) Pain is pain for a reason: The official bearer of bad tidings, its duties include shouting down, distracting, and rudely jumping in line ahead of other feelings.

What this errant questioner should have been asking was, "What are you experiencing? Setting aside the pain for a moment if you can, describe all the physical and emotional sensations that you perceive?" Is it pain, or pain's sidekick–fear? Your body respects pain as an important messenger, but deeply loathes fear. Among other responses, the body reacts to fear by radically adjusting your internal chemical mix and modifying essential cellular functions, throwing some into hyper-drive and drastically curtailing others. The objective is to urgently fortify the membranes of your cells to exclude whatever it is that is giving off the smell, the taste, the vibes, the rot of fear and possible death.

This is a good thing, but damaging if pain is allowed to override all other feelings that often provide a more comprehensive and accurate reading of your health.

No Fooling

Pain in general is not an emotion, although it evokes strong secondary emotion-like states of mind, and in the case of chronic, recurring illness can lead to panic, dread and depression, which are close cousins of fear. First and foremost, pain is a symptom of a physical condition—a form of sensory perception that announces itself in a way that is impossible to ignore. The mind has an amazing talent for converting routine physical sensations into conscious awareness that can instantly influence behavior without engaging in a formal, carefully executed, cognitive process. Courtship and mating rituals are examples. Romeo and Juliet embraced first, and only later considered the pros and cons of love. Driven mad by jealousy deviously stirred up by Yago, Othello strangled Desdemona. Likewise, random mood swings seem to come and go independently of any obvious provocation. In a flash we jump from glad to sad, from self-ishness to generosity, from calm to jittery. We slam down the phone, honk the car horn or yell at the dog. Alternatively, we don't slam, honk, or yell—choosing instead to shrug or

nod or smile. Some of us are better at managing our emotions. Managed well or poorly, the bottom line is that emotions convey many messages inspired by direct interaction
with the real world. Feelings allow us to re-experience the
experience. Emotions tend to have an honest, utilitarian and
traceable lineage.

Fear instigated by pain, however, is a bastard that lacks the
legitimacy of context. Once the sensory readout crosses the invisible threshold between mild and moderate discomfort, the
response to pain isn't modulated by reason, recollection or experience, like a relatively healthy emotion. Oh, no. It hurts,
and Fred or Judy want it to stop. The arc of escalation leaps
from "so what" to "I'm screwed."

We are going to take a close look at why this happens
and what can be easily done to recover healthy emotional
control. For now, though, it is more useful to establish the
powerful pain-fear connection, introduce how it hijacks a
fairly simple, orderly bio-mechanical sequence to set off a
chain reaction of damaging consequences. By treating pain
as just another emotional component that is always hover-
ing nearby in moments of sickness and in health, he (Mr.
How-do-you-feel I began introducing a few pages back) unintentionally condemned those he was trying to help (except
for a small minority) to the futility of symptomatic treatment, where pain escalates, where despair and disorienta-
tion set in, and where the body's amazing power to heal
itself is compromised.

"My back hurts...."

"My knee is killing me...."

"These headaches are horrible...."

What wonderful answers! I could immediately go to work
eliminating the pain. Except it was a symptom (perhaps not

even the most important symptom), rather than the actual cause of very real, ultimately life-changing and life-threatening situations.[1]

That's right—me. I asked the wrong question again and again because I knew with absolute certainty that these painful conditions could be fixed with a few simple postural remedies. By asking "How do you feel?" I really meant "I already know. Save your breath, I can fix you"—although I did not realize it at the time. I had become an 'expert', telling people what to do and how to do it. Meanwhile, I was criticizing other experts for offering remedies that substituted their knowledge and skills for the pain-sufferer's own instincts. "The patient knows best," I insisted. "Each of us knows how we feel. The Egoscue Method—my life work—delivers results because it rests on trust that stems from how the patient really feels. Those feelings are always right."

I had only one problem: I didn't believe it.

Don't worry, this book is about you, not me. I will get out of the way after presenting a bit more background; then it will be my privilege to guide you on a journey of rediscovery that can change the way you experience the rest of your life. That Joseph Campbell epigram at the top of the chapter isn't just window dressing. It is the real deal—you <u>can</u> experience the rapture of being alive.

---

[1] If you break a leg in a fall, the fracture is the cause of pain, and the pain is obviously a symptom. But if a physician manages to kill the pain the leg is still broken. Suppressing the pain symptom is relatively easy, but there is usually much more work to be done, and my point is—too often it isn't.

The Big Picture

Okay, back up three paragraphs to my first direct reference to the "Egoscue Method." As a non-medical postural therapy program, the Egoscue Method works and works quickly. Often, in less than ten or fifteen minutes there are dramatic results. A distinctive posture accompanies musculoskeletal system pain. By changing the posture, the pain diminishes significantly or abates entirely. Typically, patients are evaluated by a therapist, coached through a customized series of postural exercises, and then they are sent home to do daily workouts for a week or two. When they return to us, we expect to see a big change. As the years have gone by, I never understood what was happening when I, or one of my staff therapists, asked the opening question as the second round of in-clinic treatment began—"How do you feel right now?" We'd hear the blandest of generalities come from eighty percent of our new patients. We would get "Fine," "So-so," and my least favorite—"I don't know, you tell me."

Huh? Run that by me again. So-so? You don't know ...?

Was this the same person who could barely move ten days before? Instead of high-fives, instead of rejoicing that the pain had subsided or gone away completely after weeks and even years of suffering, there was a forgetful, guarded, almost disbelieving attitude.

Often, I had to press them to grudgingly admit that, "Yes, my back feels much better." Or, "Pain comes and goes after I do the exercises you recommended instead of hurting constantly."

I'd glance at their original intake interview and note that the pain had caused severe insomnia. "How about sleep?"

"Oh, yeah—I'm sleeping better."

I dealt with these baffling responses by telling myself that these patients were so obsessed with their pain that they were unable to look beyond the symptom and realize that by restoring their posture they felt a whole lot better in general—more energy, activity levels soaring, mobility recovered, mood improved and so on. The vast macro changes didn't register on their consciousness, and the many significant micro effects of pain abatement seemed to be quickly forgotten or severely undervalued once the hurting subsided.

"When I ask, 'How do you feel,'" I rationalized, "I'm focusing on the big picture, the *panorama* of benefits. Most people are satisfied if the pain *close-up* goes way. They want a successful treatment and that's what they got. Case closed. Move on." Never mind that the dropout rate was high (though, as a gross number of our high intake spread over several years, the percentage was a reasonable single-digit percentile, at worst), and many of those who drifted away from active therapy eventually returned to seek our help later with other incidents of pain and dysfunction; repeat business that I took as a vote of confidence in the Method.

As for the other imposing slice of my clients, what was going on there? After first experiencing short programs of postural exercises, they reported that not only had the pain eased but they could feel major changes in energy levels, mood, balance and sense of well-being. They didn't need prompting or prodding. It was the fountain of youth. They were excited and raring to do more. Frequently, it led to a total health makeover. Favorite sports and activities that had been put aside because of age or 'wear and tear' were resumed and deeply savored.

The best I could do to explain was that one group "got it" and the other didn't. I was right, but it took me a long time to figure out why.

The turning point was the realization that even I didn't get it. I was treating my own body like a machine: Keep it fueled, lubricated, put air in the tires and everything was fine. I ran, lifted weights, took vitamins and watched what I ate. After all, I was "the posture guy"; I worked conscientiously at tuning up my musculoskeletal system, and pain was not an issue. Yet there were other issues: anger, frustration, regret, fear. On one level, I could say I felt okay. On another, I felt lousy. What was my body telling me?

Meanwhile, I was forced to grapple with an alarming business trend. Starting in the mid-1990s, my growing national network of Egoscue Method clinics was retaining a smaller and smaller percentage of the clients who started with us.[2] These clients didn't behave like unhappy customers. As a result, our operating revenue and profit margins came from the largest segment of customers that by definition was receiving nowhere near the value it was paying us to provide.

I ran the numbers over and over again in disbelief: A surprisingly high percentage of my clients were dropping out of the program as soon as the pain abated, which in almost every case was way too soon to lock in fully restored musculoskeletal system functions. Our mantra was, and is, "A cure, not just treatment." Why settle for treatment when a comprehensive cure was available? They were settling for less. I started quizzing those who remained: What was motivating them to continue?

---

[2] Roughly eight to ten in-clinic therapy sessions of ninety minutes each would constitute 'full' treatment and, in most cases, a cure of the condition that brought the individual to us in the first place. In other words, our non-medical, postural therapy eliminated pain, physical limitation, and restored musculoskeletal function. Otherwise, postural therapy would continue at our expense until those results were achieved and the client fully satisfied. Less than two or three percent expressed dissatisfaction; but the actions of a silent majority—not finishing the therapy cycle—indicated there was a problem.

Slowly, the pieces fit together. One, the Egoscue Method alleviated pain without surgery or drugs. Two, being pain-free left the patient feeling healthier in general. And three, by escaping from pain and locking in musculoskeletal system realignment and strengthening their posture, those who persevered regained peace of mind and enormous self-confidence. Most importantly, what they felt sprang from their inner emotional perceptions, not from externally provoked physical sensations.

What I was looking at was a classic mind-body connection that confirmed my own personal experience: Often troubling health issues are centered in the emotions rather than in any internal, physical malfunction or shortcoming. Consequently, it seemed reasonable to embark on a close examination of major Eastern religions that have led the way for centuries in exploring how and why the body and mind interact. It has been an enlightening pathway, and I am grateful to the many helpful teachers, scholars, philosophers and friends who have guided me.

This book sets out to demonstrate that the mind-body connection is the pivot-point on which your health balances. Furthermore, years of studying the human musculoskeletal system convince me that posture functions as an on-off switch that activates emotions; through them it allows you to optimize your health without the need for increasingly common major medical intervention driven by experts, many of whom operate on the sincere but erroneous assumption that the body is fragile, makeshift and prone to break down.

When the mind-body connection is working well, and working with fully balanced posture, you directly experience the effects of your external environment—an effusion of positive, pleasurable, life-affirming emotions help regulate the mind and the body. Hence cell membranes, which I

mentioned a few pages ago, do not need armor-plating to exclude toxins. Nor is it necessary to urgently adjust our inner
chemistry by pouring hormones into the bloodstream or
dumping T-cells into combat zones of infection like so many
ninja warriors. Balanced posture amounts to an unob-
structed window. It tells us many things in real-time about
our mind-body health, not the least of which is news that
positive energy is flowing in abundance through the membrane—the "brain of the cell." The destination—actually tens
of billions of destinations—is cellular mitochondria contain-
ing enzymes that accomplish electron transport, the citric
acid cycle, and fatty acid oxidation to rejuvenate the cell
with ATP, a concoction of oxygen, heat, water and nutrients:
the equivalent of jet fuel and matzo ball soup. The cells
gorge on ATP, gobbling up and burning off the volume
equivalent of half your body weight each day. Courage,
calmness, strength and renewal flourish. The cup runneth
over, and it is on display in plain sight.

In order to survive, every form of life must stay in close
contact with its external environment and engage in constant
two-way negotiations.[3] If the environment changes abruptly—
and change is an historical certainty of living on Earth—the
organism either adapts successfully to the new circumstances
or dies. Of the 30 billion individual species of organisms believed to have existed on this planet since life first emerged,
only $1/100^{th}$ of 1% survives today. Extinction is the rule, not
the exception. Clearly, change is not easy to accomplish. It is
highly unlikely that the secret of our longevity is brain

---

[3] Colin Tudge

power—or to be more precise "prefrontal cortex power."[4] Cell power is probably more like it. Cells are classic know-it-alls. We are dummies in comparison. Each of your cells comes with a complete copy of your genetic code. In short, cells have two instruction books: one, chapter and verse on how to do its assigned specialty, and a second volume informing it on all the fine points of every other cell's specialty. Information-sharing is total. There does not appear to be a single blank spot within the body.

However, if the connection is off-kilter, that's when your posture is compromised (almost always, visibly) by imbalance and dysfunction. The arrogant, egocentric mind thinks it possesses the power to control reality by the force of intellectual firepower. Although human beings are gifted with capacity for high EQ—"emotional intelligence"[5]—bending reality to our will is an illusion. The effort brings on a dark cloud of negative emotions—thunderheads of fear, futility and anger. Why? We are in way over our heads, and know it. The frenetic, calculating 'me mind' tries to fix the internal problem when, in fact, no fixing is required. Nothing internal is broken. The cells are healthy. Even so, they are put on red alert, revved up to fight the thinking mind's illusory fears. Little by little, the defeats that come from battling the wrong enemies take a damaging toll: Health deteriorates, and the symptoms of dysfunctional posture bear silent witness to that decline.

---

[4] The brain's anterior-most lobe apparently controls executive functions like planning, goal-setting, and urge suppression.
[5] Daniel Goleman

Poor posture is a symptom—a limitation—that is being duly warned of by pain or stiffness. A drooping head, slumping shoulders, and wobbling gait (and a host of other characteristics) are confirmation that the mind is too busy sending out frantic SOS messages that it can't find the energy resources needed to keep your musculoskeletal system functions operating up to par. Eventually, it has no other choice but to ring the big gong—pain. The modern thinking mind—a term I use to distinguish it from the much older, aware, feeling mind—is a worrywart. Perpetually alarmed by the losing struggle to perfectly control reality, it bombards the body with hormonal warnings that end up reshaping our musculoskeletal system, and over- and under-revving important internal physiological processes. In turn, anxiety is stoked up even more by the musculoskeletal system's precarious condition, which can include muscular weakness, inflexibility, instability, and severe limitations of function and routine mobility.

I used to believe that by returning to good posture, the peace and balance of the aware mind would be restored simultaneously. My mistake was to regard the absence of pain as the principal requirement. By eliminating pain, I assumed people would continue to eagerly work on recovering their musculoskeletal system to full function because it felt good. I underestimated the power of the thinking mind to remain locked in crisis mode.

But why do a minority of patients escape from such a dire situation? By working closely with both groups, I can answer that question. The winners possess peace of mind securely anchored by the positive energy accessed by an aware mind, which is reinforced and even supported by a less-than-perfect posture that nevertheless is a causal source of determination and confidence.

Distilling Emotion from Experience

The first task of this book is to forge a reasonably coherent understanding of the causal link that begins with positive energy and spans good posture, good health, the aware mind and, at the same time, connects to the balanced vitality and vibrancy that come from peace of mind, which lies deep within our oldest and richest legacy as human beings.

Causality? Yeah, afraid so.

Try not to overcomplicate causality. Philosophers have long struggled to elaborate on a concept that is waterlogged with tears of frustration and exhaustion. Think of causality as a pool that holds the first droplet of human experience and the next ten billion droplets. In the beginning there was a solitary, hardly noticeable speck of moisture; now there is enough water to drown a cat (don't worry about Miss Fluffy, she does an impressive butterfly). In both cases, events occurred, reoccurred and went on to accumulate mass. Today's pool owes its existence to the first drip, the last or most recent drips and those in between. Without all of them, without the chain that stretches from one to the other, from the past to the present, that cat would be dry and purring.

There is no requirement for cats or cabbages to be aware of the individual droplets, yet consciousness of the awaiting pool is a certainty that has important consequences for the meandering cat and other passersby. Human beings have the capacity to recollect events (and to a degree, cats do too). We store them in our memory banks as event-patterns, and as such, the patterns form distinct experiences that generate meaning(s) and are organized as emotions that influence behavior. Meaning. Emotions. Behavior.

Wow, made it by hopping from rock to rock! The going got pretty slippery but here we are back to emotions.

Choose or Lose

The creation of the experiential pool is a series of events that form an experience that expresses meaning denoted by the emotions felt by those who lived through the events (e.g., Kitty hates getting her ears wet) and who are capable of periodic recollection of both the events and the emotions. Also they have power to shape past, present and future behavior. Every link in the causal chain represents the impact of energy in the form of particles or waves performing work or causing external (and internal) change. Causality is mandatory for all things. Awareness is our choice. Likewise, unawareness is too. Either way, experiences and the emotions associated with those past experiences have impact moving forward.

If this seems like what the circus clowns used to call a Chinese fire drill, give yourself a chance to digest my riff on causality. Our health and its effect on our emotions and actions are governed by a causal relationship that explains the essential intricacies of the mind-body connection that are within our power to make conscious (aware) choices. Am I saying aware choice is good? You bet I am.

When Marie first came to my Egoscue clinic in Del Mar, California, she made a choice to think of herself as an "overweight, overworked mother" of two children. Her words, not mine. She was thirty-eight years old. Her lower back hurt— big time. A physician had diagnosed the pain as a symptom of a herniated disk. From the way she stood against my office wall (her back was flat against the surface) I suspected that she had two herniated disks: The second one was just getting started.

I asked her why she elected to come to see me. She said that a friend had recommended the Egoscue Method as having a reputation for getting fast results. Marie didn't have time for pain. I explained that her spine had lost most of its lower S-curve due to years of sitting in a chair for hours at a time. Consequently, a vertebrae of the spine exerted uneven pressure on the disk and walked (i.e., nudged or levered) it out of its proper position until a nerve got in the way.

"Can I walk it back in?" she asked.

"No, but you can do the next best thing," I said.

In the first hour, we managed to eliminate about two-thirds of the pain by engaging pelvic muscles that partially restored the S-curve. In effect, we repositioned the spine and got it off the nerve. I gave her a homework menu of postural exercise that took about forty minutes a day to complete. When she left, I wondered if Marie would stick with it or opt for a much faster treatment—surgery—rather than the more time-consuming process of curing her spinal dysfunction.

Three weeks and a couple of telephone calls later, Marie was back and she had made another choice: She was no longer "overweight and overworked." Well, maybe she could lose a few pounds, but her harassed, hurry-to-be-buried attitude had changed.

"By getting rid of so much of the pain the first day and the rest a few days later, I realized that all I needed to do was restore my balance by getting aligned and my energy levels would zoom upward. I haven't felt this good in fifteen years."

Marie was relaxed and all smiles. "The results were almost instant. I can feel the energy flowing and percolating from head to foot when I start doing the E-cises."[6]

---

[6] At Egoscue Method clinics postural therapy comes in the form of "E-cises"™ that reengage, realign and strengthen musculoskeletal system functions.

I told her she had lost her deer-in-the-headlights look. Marie laughed. "Yeah, I was really freaked." What Marie did was to rediscover cause and effect. We humans are designed to engage our sensory (emotional) mechanism that links to electrochemical trace-data stored in our cells. This data has been preserved in the form of an indestructible pulse of energy. Think of it this way: You eat a candy bar as an afternoon snack. Regardless of whether you bother to read the ingredients on the wrapper, sugar, cocoa, various coloring agents, preservatives and artificial flavorings affect–stimulate–a response that is felt immediately or is stored for later. In other words, energy is obtained and used to cause change within the body or is stockpiled to make a change happen in the future.

The Virtue of Thoughtlessness

We humans know this reserved energy as emotions, feelings. If you fished the discarded candy wrapper out of the trash, you would have information about products stored in your body. Similarly, if you fished a discarded event from your memory banks, you'd find stored-up emotions or emotional subcomponents. Yet what you feel is different from what you think. A memory of an incident we experienced is produced by an electrochemical event stored in the cells as energy; when triggered, or remembered, the feeling announces its origin to the brain and the rest of the body as anger, surprise or any of a score of familiar expressions of emotion-laden energy. We don't have to think about emotion–we feel it. But if you don't know how you feel, your sensory output and perception go unheeded. Hence, making a choice–an emotionally informed choice–is impossible.

You exist today because your ancestors knew how they felt, took appropriate action, and then stored the information that allowed them to make a similar choice sometime in the future. If you don't know how you feel, beyond being assailed by powerful emotions that are pummeling all your physiological processes, you're on a tightrope without a safety net, and we better get busy putting one in place.

The time has come to restore your right to choose how you feel.

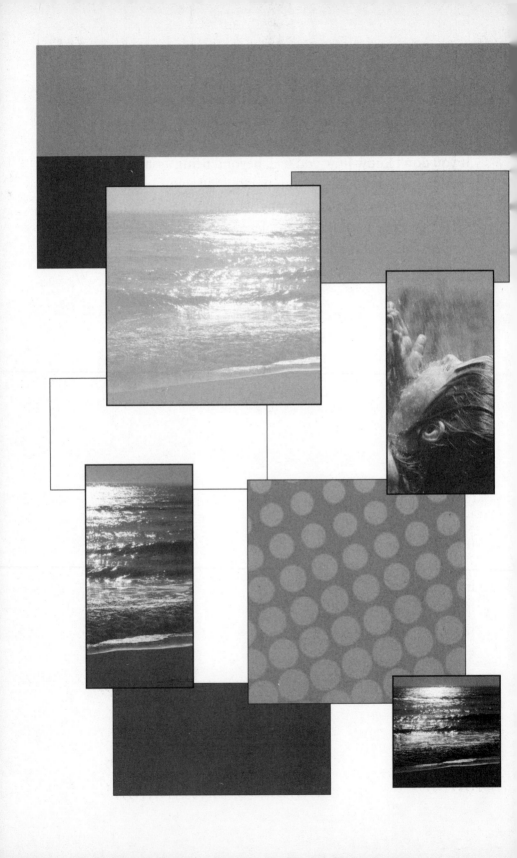

The Calm

In spite of all the testing and sophisticated scientific research associated with today's advanced medical treatment techniques, the most reliable way to promote healing and full recovery from accidents and chronic disease is to rely on the individual's awareness of how he or she feels.

Awareness. Don't worry. I'm not using the word in any special poetic or spiritual sense. This is totally basic. We can do awareness. This island of life that harbors us is full of noises, alluring scents, sharp edges, sweet tastes, and shooting stars. Our awareness is a great—quite possibly the greatest—treasure that we possess. It is a survival tool that took us from a precarious perch on a golden bough at the edge of a dark forest to a transcendence so complete there is no better choice but to close your eyes, take a deep breath and let awareness take its course.

"How are you?" is a serious question. "Fine, thank you" was the preprogrammed default answer until about a hundred years ago when medical innovation began to take off. Until then, to safeguard their health, sensible people had to rely on the body's practicality and flexibility. Things were pretty simple. All he or she needed to do was to pay attention. Sooner or later an obvious change occurred: A strong stomach turned queasy, a long distance walker started getting blisters on her feet, a hunter's acute hearing faded, and that sort of thing. In other words, they'd receive a warning featuring *symptoms* that suggested potentially harmful conditions were setting in or triggering internal alarms—spiking temperature, inflamed tissue, aching joints, and the like.

I use the word *symptoms* in italics because the health crisis we find ourselves in today started with a fundamental error involving symptoms. A symptom does not cause sickness or chronic disease. It is a calling card, a fingerprint, a signpost. Such as it is, a symptom is a sneaky and slippery operator. On the surface the word seems to define itself as a supporting actor—more adjective than a straightforward noun. In reality, symptoms have aspirations to be determinators. To do so, they exploit humankind's aptitude for thinking up and building mechanical systems; generations of engineers and the consumers of highly engineered products have been trained to replace parts that squeak, rattle, clank or freeze up. It is second nature to work back to the preceding level and so on until the symptom first appears, then resort to a hacksaw or wrench. Remove the symptom, fix the problem.

But the body isn't a machine; it is an array of incredibly intricate processes that originate inside the boundaries of the individual flesh-and-blood capsule. The hacksaw and wrench only silence the internal alarms. Soundlessly (perhaps painlessly), the real cause continues to be felt in other ways that are detrimental to health.

I promise to elaborate on my reference to 'incredibly intricate processes' as we work our way through the book. For now, stick close to cause and effect. I'm going to assume you want a cure, not just a treatment. If you can't tell me—far more importantly, can't tell yourself—how you feel, you are causeless and in a fundamental way, sense-less. When attempts at a solution to a health problem are disjointed treatments—wild pitches that inevitably get wilder and wilder.

Comparison Shopping

Okay, step off the mound for a moment. My next task is to convince you that your body is damned-near perfect. All you need to do is choose a physiological function: Digestion or respiration will do; climbing a set of stairs is awesome; or to be truly impressed, study reproduction. Spend a couple of hours in the library or on the Internet doing a little research. You will come away, I hope, with the sense that something with so many moving parts, chemical reactions and interactions, synchronicity and almost impossibly precise timing doesn't tend to make mistakes. Yes, I'm hedging a bit. Nature is not without a few flaws; cells that zigged instead of zagged. Yet it happens relatively rarely, and nowhere near as often as would be suggested by the mass media's focus on new epidemics, new diseases and new doomsday scenarios that have convinced millions of people that their damned-near perfect bodies are fragile and prone to break down.[7]

Like the brain, our other physiological processes have many alternative pathways to choose from to get around obstacles. Medical science has yet to find the exact causes of the

---

[7] Only 5% of the population is affected by gene defects (Lipton).

marquee killer diseases, like the many forms of cancer. With fewer symptomatic treatments, which are often damaging and stressful in their own right, and more attention to changing destructive inputs from outside the body, I expect many of those killers will be conquered, and it will happen soon.

Hire Up

There is just one more important task on the agenda—getting you to come back to work as CEO. You are in charge of your own health. It is up to you to decide what works, what doesn't and why. You, and you alone, are the foremost health expert.

Every human being has an incredibly sophisticated array of sensory receptors, yet the incoming messages rarely get over the threshold of conscious awareness. This is not normal; viewed across humankind's million-plus years on Earth, it is very definitely abnormal and extremely dangerous. An inverse relationship has formed with the advances in civilization, education and technological innovation, drowning out and suppressing what was once a robust stream of understandable, actionable, sensory, internal, health guidance that even an unschooled Bronze Age farmer was capable of comprehending and acting upon with a reasonably good chance of success.

Here's the plan: In the first three chapters, my top priorities are to briefly cover what has happened, why, and how you can restore your health awareness. Not a bad way to get started. It puts you in a position to take the steps necessary to reactivate an essential life-support system and resume constantly monitoring the state of your health by receiving clear warnings when there's danger, or getting positive signals in reaction to beneficial circumstances. In short order you can stop being dependent on others for health expertise.

Fire the doctor? No, of course not. Better yet, resume being the physician's working partner and best resource, the primary supplier of reliable information on the state of your own health. The doctor can make an educated guess about what's going on. You don't need to guess—you can feel it, and more than ever that's what it takes to withstand disease, accidents and premature aging.

Chapter 2 includes a simple exercise that I urge you to do without delay. Drop everything and get with it. You will feel an important change in your body and mind. The door to your perfect health will start to open.

From there we will go on to consider the musculoskeletal system's role in keeping you on an even keel, fully aware and energized. I will introduce you to the secret of humankind's evolutionary success as a species: posture. Sounds quaint, eh? Don't be fooled. Our posture announces to the world whether we are strong or weak, growing or declining, living or dying. Posture is an early warning system, the closest thing to a master key to the door to perfect health. It reacts immediately to change, sends out a cost/benefit analysis, and tells you in unmistakable terms whether you're on the right or wrong track. I'll set out three complete daily conditioning programs that will let you get on the track you decide is right for you by reengaging, strengthening and realigning your magnificent musculoskeletal system. You get to select which program works best and feels best. Not only is this the means to living pain-free without toxic drugs and traumatic surgery, it is the foundation of a long lifetime of good health in general.

Lastly, I'll share with you my understanding of the health role played by positive energy. Chronic pain is a symptom of correctable energy deprivation, not human frailty. Luckily, so is poor posture. What's lucky about it is that posture is visible and can be easily realigned from a dysfunctional state to a functional, positive, energy-generating mode. Good posture is not solely a matter of aesthetics or personal beauty. It is "good" simply because it feels good, and in that way it is a crucial element in the health-awareness feedback system that I'll be discussing.

Also coming up–a smattering of Quantum physics, Zen spiritual practices and doctrine, and assorted cutting-edge hypothesizing (like the Law of Attraction, mindfulness, David R. Hawkins' work on the beneficial power of high wavelength energy, and Bruce H. Lipton's book *The Biology of Belief*).

This is a good place to get back to the pathway we were on a few pages ago before I veered off for the overview. Today modern science, medical science in this case, has diligently claimed responsibility for all but the most superficial aspects of our health. Only a fully licensed, impressively credentialed expert need reply to such questions as 'How do you feel?' Or so it seems. The body is just too complicated for average folks to comprehend. Or so it seems.

I have a feeling that down deep you don't buy that, and you're absolutely right not to. The book you are reading is a celebration of our perfect

---

Sense and Sensibility

There are five traditional senses–sight, hearing, smell, touch and taste. Six others are also generally recognized, among them balance, awareness of time, sensitivity to temperature and pain. I believe there are many more, each supported by a sensory system that responds to specific physical stimuli. We are consciously aware of only a few. However, if we could assign a *click* to every incoming stimulus and a *clack* to the outgoing response, there would be a deafening uproar of traffic. Along with the metabolic process, sensory reception and perception may well be the essential operational cornerstone of human biology.

health, and an invitation to retrieve the body's power to heal, to grow, to live a long, joyful life free of limitations and chronic pain.

You and I, and the rest of the human tribe know more about our individual health, how we feel and why we feel it than all the so-called experts combined. That *knowing* is a gift, a legacy that has allowed humankind to do the impossible by establishing a foothold on this remote speck of the cosmos. Relinquishing such a heritage is unthinkable, yet we are under growing pressure to hand it over to those who sincerely believe themselves to be better informed and better equipped. I'm not bashing doctors or knocking big pharmaceutical companies; the blame game is a waste of time and energy. My objective is to reestablish the legitimacy of *How do you feel?* And to once again receive a direct, candid answer—not how does the cardiologist or the director of research at Merck think you feel—to a question has more salience than any other you could ask about your health.

Why? Because once you are fully in touch with how you feel, you'll know the right thing to do. Even so, one of the central themes that we will be exploring is this: Your body is smarter than you are.

Whoops! Do we need to slam on the brakes and decide where the body stops and where you start? Let's not. For now, proceed as though the physical body and the *you-mind* (i.e., a stuffy though useful shorthand for individual consciousness and cognition) are separate entities—they're not, but taking a shortcut here will save time and trouble.

Anyway, the smart body knows when it is sick, knows what it takes to get well, knows how to live a long and happy life. But the body is not omnipotent; it needs a little help from you. Your job is to pay attention and become aware of how the body is constantly changing as it responds to its environment and, when necessary, take appropriate action to support that response.

Equipped with two eyes, two ears, two hands, two feet and at least five senses, you take care of interacting with the extremely variable external environment. In return, the body keeps you informed as to what it needs to have done for it to maintain internal equilibrium, such as adequate food, water, sleep, shelter, companionship, fun and the like. If you are inattentive, don't care or prefer to pass the buck to someone else, be prepared to suffer the consequences—pain is one way the body communicates serious information. In the end, by ignoring the body's wisdom you are damaging your health and shortening your life.

You are the only one with total access to, literally speaking, complete inside knowledge on what's really happening to your physiological processes, your organs, your tissues, your cells. The body keeps you completely informed. Medical doctors can make assumptions, drug companies can research, test, and sell reasonably effective products; only you have the actual *feel* for what works and what doesn't. It is a talent, a genius you were born with.

If you opt out of playing this important role, your health is in jeopardy. The increasingly complex technology and head-spinning treatment choices make it seem like a losing battle to even think that you are such a key part of your own health.

Confusing?—sort of.

Challenging?—sure.

"Losing"?—never!

All you need is to be reconnected to the power of perfect health that comes from taking action, making choices based on knowing the answer to a simple four-word question:

How do you feel?

I know that you know—now let's explore that knowing together.

Balancing Act

If you've read any of my four previous books, you may remember that I like to encourage the reader to participate in the fun and games. Well, here I go again.

Take off your shoes and socks.

And stand up. Please.

If you are driving a car and listening (I hope you're not reading and driving!)—pull over, stop, take off your shoes and socks, get out and stand up.

In the library or a bookstore? People are giving you funny looks as you remove your socks, aren't they? Better go home before you get arrested.

All set? Read the rest of this paragraph, then shut your eyes and follow the instructions. And here they are: Stand normally, relax; let your feet, shoulders and head go where they want to go (and do go when someone isn't barking out orders). Keep your feet in place, inhale and exhale a couple of times. Take your time. Notice how your weight is distributed. One leg may be working harder than the other. Is it the right leg? Left? Feel where the weight settles in the feet— heels? Inside edge, outside edge, toward the toes? It's likely to be in a different spot in each foot. Let two or three minutes go by. Breathe.

Now, open your eyes. Read some more. Did you notice what was going through your mind when you were analyzing the weight distribution? Was there a jumble of ideas, images, and sensations? A little of this and that? Quick arrhythmic bursts of mental activity? A sensory jig-saw puzzle with a bunch of missing pieces? At the end of this paragraph, close your eyes again and pay attention to your mental traffic. Give it a minute and reopen your eyes.

Now I'd like you to balance your weight distribution evenly. Read this paragraph and close your eyes again. Edge both feet around until they're roughly parallel, pointing straight ahead and about hips-width apart. Now, turn them inward a little, till they are slightly pigeon-toed. Easy does it. Carefully swing your torso, shoulders and head around until you can feel the weight move in your feet. Did you ever play flashlight tag as a kid? The beam of light moved like a disk, didn't it? The weight will have the same characteristic: It will focus and slide here and there. Nudge the disks into the balls of your feet. Bob a little at the knees, tweak your hips. Some people will really have to crank themselves around. It may feel strange, precarious. Believe me, though, when the weight rests over the balls of the feet, your posture is in a balanced position. (The contortions and muscular effort to hold you there are necessary because your musculoskeletal structure is fighting to pop out of the temporary alignment that I've put you in.) When you get the weight centered, notice how it feels, notice what your mind is doing. Go ahead, try it.

When we have clients perform the same exercise in one of our Egoscue Method clinics, most of them say that in the first unbalanced position their minds are whirling, jumpy and chaotic. They feel troubled, uncertain, uneasy. Balanced, however, is a different story. The mind calms down. It loses the jittery quality. There's more steadiness and clarity.

By changing your posture you've changed your mind. The result is similar to switching channels on a radio or TV set. A distant signal wavers and breaks up; adjusted to a closer, stronger frequency the transmission sharpens and settles down.

Am I saying that the thought process changes too? The calming, clarifying effect that people report indicates that that is probably happening. If the medium is the message, our brains are providing a smoother, less hassled ride (the defini-

> ## Vis viva ("Living Force")
>
> You are 100% energy. All matter, from rocks to race horses, is permutations of energy. Consequently, you are indestructible because energy cannot be destroyed. Forms do change, though. For instance, Shakespeare has been dead for about 400 years, yet all of his energy is still around. There is a chance that some of it may be incorporated into your corporal being—part of an ear lobe or skin tissue. Matter-energy is infinitely recyclable. Prior to residing within the thumb of the Bard's right hand, matter-energy could have been a freckle on King Tutankhamen's chin.
>
> No one knows how energy gets channeled into a particular form or how to positively distinguish between a genius' energy and that of an earthworm. In its vast variety, energy is the cosmic equivalent of chicken soup—a delicious cure-all elixir; just don't ask what's in your bowl. There's enough energy packed into the average adult human to explode with the force of thirty large hydrogen bombs (7×10^{18} joules of potential energy, according to Bill Bryson, whom I'm trusting to get it right since a calculation like that is several hydrogen bombs' worth of intellectual firepower beyond my meager capabilities), but so far we are able to release only a tiny percentage of it in one burst.

tion of a medium is a carrier, a conveyance). By not skidding on icy patches or by avoiding clunking into potholes, our whole physiological state is more tranquil, less stressed, better grounded. In short, we *feel* better.

So, standing around with eyes closed playing a form of flashlight tag with your postural weight distribution is a big deal?

Actually it is.

What you've just done is bridge the gap between mortality and immortality. Yes, that's right—immortality, for we are more than flesh and blood, more than skin and bones. We are energy. Our understanding of physics tells us that energy is indestructible.

The exercise gives us a window on the process that makes all human beings as indestructible as a block of granite. Of course, granite can be and is ground into sand over the long haul, and eventually the grains of sand are reduced to molecules of matter. Because all matter is energy, those molecules are destined to return to the vast power surge of waves and particles created by the Big Bang, where they bump and grind, pulse and pummel, push and pull across an infinity of space and time.

What our version of flashlight tag reveals is that we are not passive bystanders at the cosmic energy Olympics, but that our mortal bodies are designed to deliberately tap into and draw from the vast supply of energy to fuel our health. Furthermore, we now know how to do it–and it's easy!

If achieving postural balance calms the mind, it is reasonable to assume it also beneficially affects our other physiological systems; all of them. And that is precisely my assumption and the assumption of this book. On my weekly radio show[8], I was fond of torturing the listeners by singing bits and pieces of the old gospel song *Them Bones* –"the knee bone's connected to the thigh bone, the thigh bone's connected to the hip bone ...," and so on. The musculoskeletal system's connections extend from head to foot. The circuitry wires together the whole body and, what's more, links it to a vast field of high wavelength energy that radiates from one end of the Cosmos to the other (except that most physicists believe the Cosmos, or whatever you choose to call it, has no beginning and no end).

Keep in mind that increased mass contributes to resistance, drag, friction and heat. Heat is a variety of radiation,

---

[8] Now a weekly Internet radio show: Pain Free Radio.

and radiation affects molecular movement. Also, mass is a function of structural form, and forms vary in the way mass is expressed, from thin and readily permeable to dense and impermeable. This range is found in the human musculoskeletal system—from functional and balanced (energy-permeable) to dysfunctional and unbalanced (energy-impermeable).

Plug and Play

To visualize the role of the musculoskeletal system using an everyday analogy, think about how your TV set is connected to its power source: cord→plug→wall outlet→household wiring→electricity pole→electrical grid, and so on. If you were to step on the plug end of the TV's power cord—really tromp on it—the prongs of the plug would probably bend to the point that they'd no longer fit tightly into the wall outlet. The TV wouldn't work. Or the plug might make a loose connection that would cause the set to flicker on and off.

Your musculoskeletal system is a plug; i.e., a connector and conduit to the universal energy supply. The strength of that connection—the total volume of the incoming flow of energy—depends on postural balance. In other words, energy flow is determined by the way mass is arranged by structure. The more balanced you are, the more energy moves with less friction along the conduit and through the plug. Those who are fully balanced are receiving an unrestricted flow of high wavelength energy (there are fewer obstructions in the mind and body). Minor imbalance means that the energy inflow is only slightly impeded. But a person with severe imbalance, who is stooped, head down, shoulders rounded forward, feet shuffling and with drastically limited movement, is losing out on almost all of the available high wavelength energy.

The plug is barcly making contact, his "TV set" is flickering and about to go dark.

By being balanced to slightly off-balance, there is a steady flow of almost all the energy needed to lead an active, deeply satisfying life. Those who are badly out of balance are on the brink of shutting down. Their physiological systems, from the innermost organs to the outermost bones, muscles and joints, are collapsing.

At one time, possibly as recently as seventy to a hundred years ago, most people were in postural balance or close to it. At least that's how they appear in old photographs. Where balance was less than perfect, it was largely intact and capable of rebounding with relatively minor adjustments in activity levels. Theirs was an environment that required motion. Routine, everyday, musculoskeletal movement brought them closer to balance without much deliberate effort. Today, for a majority of the population of the economically advanced regions of the world, balance is on the wane as the high-tech environment demands less and less motion. At the same time, and not at all coincidentally, there is a growing health crisis. Medical costs are soaring, the news media regularly panics about new 'epidemics,' and severe chronic pain and lost mobility are becoming commonplace along with drastically invasive treatment techniques.

I'm concerned, but not worried—and you shouldn't worry either. Human health is a well-marked, two-way street that can take us to a long, deeply satisfying life free of chronic pain, limitation and fear—if we make a relatively simple, straightforward commitment to retaining and sustaining our legacy of postural balance. We can travel in the wrong direction on that two-way street, and we are. Presently, humankind is losing postural balance and underlying health, but what is lost can be found again. I believe we'll turn this around quickly once we put our minds—our aware minds—to it. That's the lesson of the exercise that I've shared with you in this chapter. Please try it again, and share it with your family and friends.

The starting place to a quick turnaround is to recognize that the body's amazing arrangement of muscles, bones and nerves made an important contribution to our development as a species, defines us as individuals and has a major, major, major influence on our overall health and happiness.

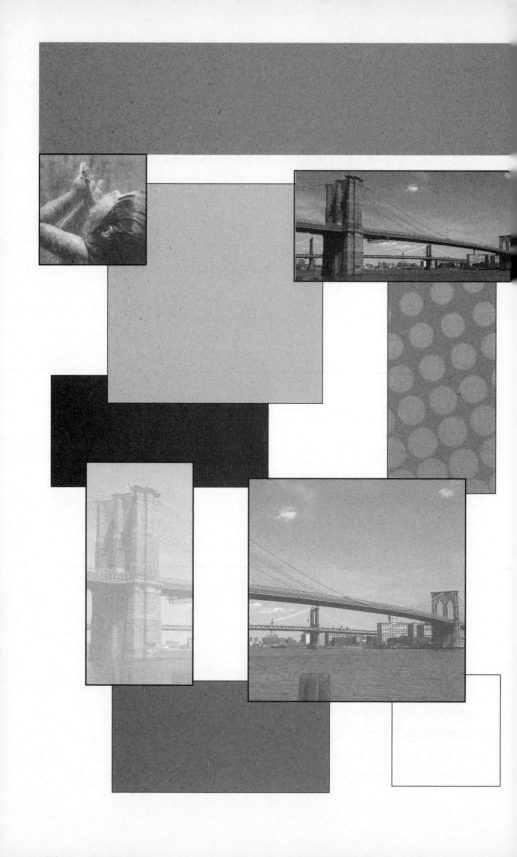

Your Fuel Gauge

Not that I'm bragging, but I don't look my age—and neither do you. Both of us are 13.7 billion years old, give or take 200 million.*

We are built to last, literally constructed out of debris: space junk, to be blunt. You and I have the good fortune to be nothing less than 100% energy produced at the creation of the universe.

Who we are varies from person to person; what we are is the ultimate in basic material. Energy is—just is; doesn't grow, procreate, subdivide or pop out of a magic lamp. It simply exists, neither being newly concocted nor in danger of being destroyed. Energy can move from place to place (or remain in place), and be changed from one form to another. In the process, it performs work, exclusively as motion or movement. You—in a non-you configuration without an ego, a face lift, and a fashionable ZIP Code—will always exist, always be on the move, always be at

*In the Beginning

Creation has become a loaded word. Created when, by whom or what? God, the Big Bang, the teeny, tiny bubbles or whatever—take your pick. Choose the Big Bang and the age of the universe is estimated to be about 14 billion years when what scientists call a "singularity" (finite matter so dense it compacted down into infinitely dense matter) suddenly exploded.

The Bubble universe is a variation that attempts to account for the pre-bang existence of so-called infinitely dense matter derived from finite matter. Basically, a foam or froth stirred up by energy fluctuation in a parent universe formed a tiny bubble that grew until it accumulated enough matter to spin off galactic structures and eventually life-forms, either before or after a sudden, huge expansion.

The bubble and bang process probably adds another 15 billion years or more to the age of our universe (it is guesswork, however, since all we see, thanks to astronomer Edwin Hubble, is the evidence of the Big Bang in the form of relatively proportional expansion that appears to come from one flash point or event). As for God, the theologians have their own timelines beginning with the Torah that puts the age of the universe at 5,758 years.

work (unless you do time as stored or *potential* energy, and then you'll get a break from work until you become kinetic energy again).

Like the ghost in Richard Wagner's opera *Der Fliegende Holländer*–a Dutch sea captain doomed to sail forever, with time off only once every seven years to find the love of a good a woman to share his fate–you are in the same boat (without the love loophole).

Basically, you are on a very long voyage. If immortality does not appeal–can't live without your Blackberry–how about 80, 90, 100 years or more of perfect health as an added attraction? Energy tosses the whole idea of chronic disease and aging right out the window. Energy doesn't get sick or old. Energy moves, yet it has no moving parts like those of a clock or an internal combustion engine, no sprockets and levers that can wear out or break. Instead, energy has various expressions, some working one way, such as digesting breakfast to stoke the cellular ATP boiler that converts the bacon and eggs into adenosine 5'-diphosphate, the metabolic fuel used to power the body's cells[9]; others are busy repairing your stockpile of various specialized proteins, perhaps 20,000 per cell which undergo heavy wear and tear from handling basic tasks like muscular contraction and respiration. Nothing is broken, diseased or wrong; energy is merely on the move, doing work amidst various anatomical and physiological structures—work that includes building, maintaining and animating those structures, as well as having been involved in creating them in the first place. A constant interplay of action and reaction takes place as particles, waves, forces and force fields carom off one another; become ripples, torrents and tsunami; raise and lower temperatures; set fires, and trigger chemical reactions and combinations that even the maddest of mad scientists couldn't dream up.

Close Resemblance

I am going to use a pocketful of metaphors to explain what happens.

Matter tends to be both pushy and sticky. By 'pushy,' I mean that it can use the equivalent of head-butts to abruptly alter the status quo. Particle energy collides with or zooms past slow-moving matter (and sometimes slips around loosely packed molecules and runs straight through without making contact), which tends to bring on a quick, dramatic reorganization of the neighborhood. Imagine a toddler

---

[9] Stedman's Medical Dictionary

pouncing into the middle of a flock of feeding pigeons. To understand 'sticky,' dig out your notes from first-year college physics: Objects that have mass attract one another; the more mass, the more attraction. Congratulations, you were paying attention.

Gravitational attraction glues newly arriving energy to existing matter and can, layer by layer, bring about a complex composite of many different forms of matter that are capable of slowly (or suddenly) transforming a stagnant puddle (matter in its earliest stages probably lodged in ocean sediment) into a chowder teeming with life. Billions of years of push and stick churned up (or shuffled) these ingredients, while extreme temperatures and pressure helped synthesize nucleic acid that allowed amino acids to produce protein combinations that jump-started single-cell life forms.

There is another important concept to be put on the table: Like attracts like. Energy vibrates by moving through space in zigs and zags like the teeth of a serrated steak knife. There are sharp peaks and narrow valleys. The steeper and deeper the declivities, the more potent the energy. In other words, the blade is sharper in that the total surface area of the cutting edge is longer and moves faster and more efficiently. There may be hundreds more peaks, descents, valleys and ascents. Now reach for another helping of gravity sauce—ultra-high wavelength energy zooms past low wavelength energy because the mass of the sluggish resident energy has negligible gravitation attraction. It may twitch or throb but doesn't solidly bond to the incoming energy. Its mass is too spongy. Alas, no sticky … no likey … no changey.

All forms of life prosper or perish as a result of an ability to make productive use of the work generated by this swirl of energy. The failure rate is high. Eventually every thing that lives dies—yet energy couldn't care less. It is here, there and everywhere to stay. Meanwhile, extinction—the wholesale elimination of particular life forms—seems to be in the cards. In the short run, as I pointed out in Chapter 1, less than 1/100th of 1% has made the cut since life on Earth began about four billion years ago. There have been millions (one estimate is 30 billion) of now-you-seem-them-now-you-don't species, many lasting seconds and a relatively few others holding on for centuries. Today, estimates of the number of living species of plants, insects, animals and "organic others" (not counting all the tiniest of the tiny multitude of micro-organisms) range upward from five to thirty million. The as-yet-undead have been extraordinarily, and improbably, lucky to have lasted so long.[10]

The casualties all lost the ability to change internally, a non-negotiable requirement that allows for the continual accommodation of the fluctuating external flow of incoming energy. For a while, reproduction and hereditary gene transfer go on, though it is more than likely that the processes are gradually compromised until systemic equilibrium and viability weaken and collapse.

The premature ageing and death of an individual are similar to the extinction of an entire species. John, for instance, was a high-powered Washington lobbyist who, in his twenties and thirties, managed the stress produced by his demanding professional life by running every morning and hitting the gym for workouts several times a week. He loved his routine—for good reason. Incoming energy (stress, including fatigue, cellular damage and other ramifications) was counteracted by the release of internal energy stored in the muscles, which boosted John's heart rate, metabolism, and cell replacement cycle. He was balancing both the incoming and outgoing flow of energy. The regular intense workouts flushed away debris and damage

---

[10] Bryson

caused by stress and the real world's hard knocks using incoming external energy to release energy stored in the muscles to rev up metabolic activity, elevated heart rate and increased respiration. In other words, by working out regularly John deliberately made an internal change take place. His physiological systems were working smoothly in balance. Yet, for some reason–'too busy' is the usual suspect–he started cutting back on running and visits to the gym. Gradually, there was more incoming stressful change and less internal balancing change. Cells died at a higher and higher rate, their efficiency declined, and subtle alterations of all of his physiological processes took place. John started to feel the effects so he resorted to vodka to adjust his internal chemistry. Drinkers think they are imbibing to make merry or to unwind, yet what they are actually doing is desperately fiddling with their body fluids. Ethanol is matter; hence, it is energy. However, not much work is accomplished other than quickly altering mood and, more insidiously, interfering with oxygen intake, blood composition and liver function. As a result, stress got the upper hand. The cumulative imbalance from incoming change swamped John's health. He died of colon cancer at the age of fifty-two.

Last Resort

This book is going to show you that millions of women and men like John prematurely age, sicken and die because their health loses balance and is unable to bring about routine internal changes that once took place in the course of daily life. Historically, when bad weather wiped out an important food crop, business as usual came to a halt: people migrated, ate grasshoppers, or plundered their neighbors. When all else failed, they starved. Change–behavioral change–was imperative and they knew it. Even so, some changes are out of reach. A gigantic dust cloud kicked up by a meteor the size of Times Square that slammed into the Earth probably doomed large dinosaurs by blotting out the sun's rays. The voracious reptiles were unable to change their internal requirement for readily available calories found in the tropical swampland as plants or in the protein of the flesh of smaller, plant-eating creatures.

Adios, T. Rex. But other forms of life did change and survive. In such cases, a change in behavior was involved. While John changed by giving up running and workouts, he was really acting like a giant, bad-tempered reptile with a tiny brain. He kept stressing his body, provoking the need for internal change, and stopped providing precisely the kind of behavioral response that accomplishes the necessary internal change. Why? Not stupidity. My answer is that John allowed himself to be distracted by a modern lifestyle that drowns out the most essential messages delivered by his senses—e.g., important news flashes: *This feels good, keep it up! That feels bad, stop right now!*

Not only was John smart enough to know that running and reasonably strenuous and varied regular physical workouts were the right things to do, his posture supplied graphic evidence just in case he was not thinking straight, not receiving the sensory messages. The stiff joints and short-windedness he experienced after giving up his exercise routine were handwriting on the wall, but he misread them. They were signs all right, although not of aging.

Nature rewards efficiency and punishes inefficiency. Gathering infirmity for weeks, months and years is colossally inefficient. What is the point of wasting valuable resources—food, fresh water, and shelter—on someone who is weak and soon headed for the grave? On the contrary, sudden death by way of accidents and plagues of virulent disease are far more rational in that the fewer mouths to feed, the better. Logic strongly suggests, therefore, that humans were built for a very long life or a very short one. Cosmetic surgeons may scoff, but facial wrinkles do not mean that the end is near; however, a dysfunctional, collapsing musculoskeletal system usually does. Posture is the equivalent of the gasoline gauge in the dashboard of a car. A quick glance revealed to our early ancestors who among them was fit to fight, fit to bear and nurture children, and fit to work hard enough to prosper in the face of adversity.

John could feel his good health draining away. He could see it as well. Unfortunately, the lobbyist who never forgot a face couldn't remember what his deteriorating posture meant. Just as a building verges on collapse when its load-bearing floors and walls slump, tilt and buckle, the musculoskeletal system that loses its horizontal and vertical structures is teetering on the edge of disintegration. Without symmetrical muscular support our essential, gravity-defying, 90-degree angles give way, leaving the head, shoulders, hips and knees wobbling, grinding and gyrating until smooth, strong, spontaneous movement becomes more and more difficult. When posture stops being fully erect, squared-off, balanced, flexible, aligned side-to-side and from front to back, when it goes from being well supported by strong muscles from head to foot to a rambling improvisation of twitches, lurches and stumbles, the entire physiological package is red-lining. Breathing is compromised, the heart works harder, the colon struggles. Everything gets disrupted.

John regarded his slow-motion, cataclysmic collapse as a natural consequence of living a mere three or four decades. His unschooled ancient ancestors would have looked at a brother or sister in the same condition and begun setting aside firewood for a funeral pyre.

The Objectivity Myth

As a community, humankind has been getting smarter, more knowledgeable, even wiser about our energy heritage, but it has taken more than 7000 years. As early as 5000 BC, spiritual practitioners in what we today call India recognized that *Prana*, a form of energy, an invisible and powerful life-force, is a central causal fact of existence. Notice, I didn't say the gurus 'discovered' or 'invented' *Prana*. Human beings, ancient and modern, inherently know and trust energy because they can feel its vitality without intermediation or indoctrination, and are capable of full awareness of its gifts. From time to time, however, thinking minds—possessed of a tendency to upstage the feeling mind—set out to dethrone energy on the grounds that it is not objective.

If your mother says she loves you, Western science demands proof in the form of carefully defined, observable standards of verification that remain true in all cases without resorting to opinion, biases and emotion. In God we trust (and even that's a little dodgy), all others pay cash in the form of cold, hard facts, even if those facts clash with personal experience and gut instinct. In other words, the *objectivists* have gone outside of themselves by ignoring the feel (the personal emotional content) of what's being directly experienced and, instead, attempt to evaluate it by secondhand criteria endorsed and prescribed by committees of researchers.

From about the mid-17th century to the early to mid-20th century, Western society was hung up on using a clock or some other intricate mechanical contraption as a model—an *object* serving as an *objective* standard—to explain how most things worked, including human health. At the apogee of this period, Newtonian science looked at the world and saw the equivalent of an elaborate construct of whirring sprockets, wheels within wheels, springs that sprang and levers that lifted—all governed by laws and forces of mechanical interaction that could be plotted mathematically and summoned to

> **Brainiac**
>
> Isaac Newton, 1642-1727, formulated the law of gravitation. Newton's *The Mathematical Principles of Natural Philosophy* is widely regarded as the most influential book ever written. It showed how a universal force, gravity, applied to all objects in all parts of the Universe, and it also formulated the three laws of motion.
>
> Newton laid the groundwork for classical mechanics, the basis of modern engineering. Despite his argumentativeness, he was far and away the leading scientist in Britain and Europe by the late 1600s.

explicate (objectively) the deepest of mysteries.[11] Seen from this perspective, the world is the sum total of its many component parts; to understand any complex natural phenomenon all you have to do is take it apart and keep taking the parts apart until you come to the smallest bits of matter, which behave predictably based on their position in space, their mass and velocity.

What the Newtonians didn't count on was that small just keeps getting smaller. In due course, Quantum physicists detected matter so minuscule it behaved not like a clock, but like something that had the feel—a highly subjective feel—of energy: entangled beams of light, swarms of molecular fragments, and torrents of disobedient subatomic matter that defy objective science by acting like waves when they are supposed to be particles, and acting like particles when the Newtonian instruction manual calls for waves. Eventually, matter shrank until it entirely disappeared in one location and instantly reappeared thousands of miles away, challenging Albert Einstein's contention that nothing travels faster than the speed of light. Predictability went out the window; Quantum theorists started concocting theories

---

[11] Newton was not necessarily a Newtonian—he was way too smart for that. The clock metaphor would probably have struck him as simple-minded. Lesser mortals needed an intellectual crutch to understate what the great man meant by terms like acceleration, velocity, friction, position and the like.

that they admitted couldn't be proven and were probably certifiably daft.

Suddenly, *Prana* didn't seem so crazy after all. However, mainstream medical science is not there yet. The idea remains that the body is a clock—a malfunctioning Timex in need of an expert watchmaker to make it keep on ticking. Why? One reason is that human beings are superb toolmakers. Micro-medicine, whether it is diagnostic, surgical, or pharmaceutical, thrives on new tools. Since the invention of the hammer and the wheel, we have employed new tools to extend our control of the environment and to reshape reality. Like Archimedes' lever and fulcrum, our innovative tools move the world by doing what had once been impossible. The notion that fixing or replacing defective body parts is the way to health took hold very slowly because it seemed both impossible and unnecessary.

The first steps in that direction came as a result of humankind's tool-making talents: A reduction in the amount of movement involved in an hour's or a day's work, but without the usual penalty for sitting on one's rump; i.e., without starvation. Gradually, there was less walking, stooping, carrying loads, climbing, vigorous hand-and-arm engagement,

> **Health Awareness**
>
> Sleeping when we are tired, eating when we are hungry, and subtly modifying our diets to counteract nutritional deficiencies (a summer of leaner fish in the place of winter's fatter red meat) are vestiges of our subconscious, instinctive, self-adjusting health awareness.
>
> Electricity disrupted sleep patterns. And those who make processed food and beverages have learned how to override this innate wisdom by manipulating the sensory perception of what goes into our mouths. Excessive amounts of salt, fats, sweeteners are shamelessly used to trick people into making unhealthy choices. Widespread obesity is not an illness—it is evidence of a crime. Does that mean I think we should lock up all the evil food processors? No. We need to stop eating their harmful products.

Knock, Knock

Physicians are probably dumped on more than any other elite profession, with the exception of lawyers. Even so, there is a large reservoir of respect left over from an earlier era when the kindness of men with a black bag—and a smaller number of women, many of them mid-wives—epitomized health care. The affection for these likeable, empathetic, less-is-more medicos lives on as nostalgia for the old-time country doc whose most powerful medicines were his listening skills, gentle common sense and patience.

and the rest of a physical repertoire that had once taken men, women and children through a full range of motion each day. In its place came an ever-more-settled, ever-more-prosperous, tool-making culture, with each new generation quietly losing small though vital amounts of musculoskeletal system balance.

And what happens when balance goes? Less energy is available to grow, maintain and sustain the body; physiological systems are under more and more stress; chronic health problems multiply, and the instinctive awareness of the body's health needs is drowned out by fear.

After many years, fear eventually opened the door to New-tonian medical science becoming the dominant Western health care model: The toolmakers joined forces with the watchmakers. Fearful, running low on energy thanks in part to rapid urbanization and the first waves of the economy's shift to massive industrialization, the thinking minds of our human ancestors prevailed over the feeling minds. They began to think the body was made up of smaller and smaller parts that were prone to breaking down like all machines. If experts were needed to build, run and repair the mechanical marvels that moved freight, milled grain and loomed textiles, it followed logically that experts were needed to rebuild, repair and run the human health machine. Non-experts stepped aside to allow those with specialized knowledge and training in *objective* medical science to take over. Thus did once-lowly shamans and herbalists, midwives and barbers, tinkers, alchemists and quacks evolve into respected, wealthy, licensed members of the ruling elite.

Newtonian Overlap

For a time, the new tools and the new procedures they spawned coexisted with human awareness. Doctors were in short supply; the average person rarely saw one. And why bother? The body's own predisposition to cure and care for itself prevailed more often than not, and the placebo effect helped save many who otherwise would have been killed by bumbling apprentices. As trial-and-error experience accumulated, crude, superficial and relatively benign medical technology was wielded by many kind and prudent men and women who knew better than to risk overly drastic treatment. They gave medicine a good name. But as medical practitioners learned how to control pain, blood loss and infection, the techniques grew bolder and more invasive. By the mid-19th century a quick march was underway toward a dominant and domineering Newtonian model.

At the same time, manual labor, which for thousands of years had been the primary means of providing food, shelter and the other basic necessities of life, suddenly gave way to crafts based on tools that reduced and eventually eliminated the need for sustained physical movement, strength and endurance by offering mechanical leverage to do the hard work of digging, plowing, reaping, lifting, carrying, weaving and building cottages or castles. A shovel, for instance, is a hand tool—and a high-tech one in its first days—that helped the hands dig deeper holes faster. But powerful muscles and coordination were still essential. A steam shovel does the digging while the operator sits and moves levers and foot peddles. Fewer (and different) muscles are involved; the close interaction of joints, nerves and physiological process, including metabolism and respiration, changes in minor and major ways.

Until the Industrial Revolution, manpower and woman-power did the work (in other words, the movement of the human body produced energy). In just a few decades, technology changed that and liberated humankind from drudgery and started a deconditioning process that has drastically affected human health. Urbanization and industrialization have eliminated at least fifty percent of the muscular and skeletal movement that was once routine. Overcrowding and primitive conditions were indeed factors in causing outbreaks of disease like the plague, but those who settled in the emerging urban areas of the world were threatened by another scourge—lack of motion.

This 'objective' version of medical science, built upon Sir Isaac's amazing mathematical acrobatics, is bankrupting us.

By chasing after smaller and smaller physiological components, systems and processes deemed to be diseased and defective, the latter-day Newtonians set off an explosion of costly medical technology that promises to make the care it offers us as unaffordable as it dangerous. Your body, ever aware, even if your thinking mind is not, is still trying to make itself heard.

War and Peace

What I am suggesting—but you know more than I do—is to feel your way toward musculoskeletal system balance, move away from objectivity, away from the broken clock. I believe you can do it because I have done it myself and now know the incredible peace of mind of perfect health. I have helped many other people make the same journey.

The very fact that you are still reading this book indicates that you are evaluating my message by the feel of it rather than the think of it. In terms of the thinking mind, Newton has me beat. He was a brilliant conceptualizer and abstract thinker. But your body is even smarter. It won't let you die without fully deploying its genius for survival.

I almost wrote "It won't let you die without a fight." I don't feel comfortable with health-as-warfare similes. The body is far too wise to seek war; it goes to peace, peace of mind—a state that can be achieved only by postural balance.

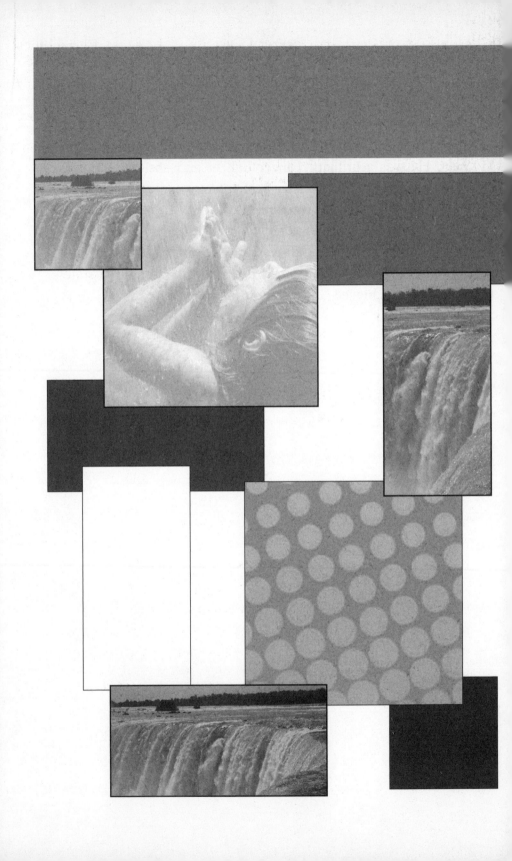

Fear & Limitation

So, how do you feel?

Take a moment to think about it; better yet, put thinking aside and be *aware* of how you feel. By distorting what is actually being experienced due to the habit of assigning largely arbitrary values to what we have seen, touched, tasted, heard and smelled, the thinking mind can prevent an accurate reading of your feelings. It's not necessary to minutely scrutinize, measure or judge what's going on. Just notice; pay attention without imposing meaning, judging or coming to conclusions. Accept that your senses are busily soaking up stimuli without making value judgments. Find this incoming stream and let it go to work on your perceptions. In due course, you'll rediscover how to distinguish the meaningful high-energy input from the meaningless background noise of second-guessing and casual censoriousness.

On Your Mind

Conscious thought—storing, retrieving and prioritizing experiences, including secondhand experiences, with the explicit goal of solving a problem or influencing an outcome—is probably no more than fifty or sixty thousand years old as a common human trait. Prior to that it seems likely that conscious thought was basic memory retrieval. Remembering is an important survival skill: where's the best nesting, the safest migration routes and the like. A few of our ancestors were able to tag what they remembered with something extra, emotion. They could re-experience an event by recalling how it felt. This conferred an enormous evolutionary advantage by mingling memory and motivation.

Once you have located the feeling, describe it. Be both general and specific. If there is pain, is it tenderness or tightness? Does the pain move around or change in intensity? Does it seem to come from muscles, nerves or joints? Summarize with a word or two: *concentrated*; *weak*; *sluggish*; *intermittent*; whatever. *Don't know* may be a cop-out. Sometimes it can be an honest reading, yet usually it means *I know but I don't want to face up to reality; hiding out in dreamland is more comforting*. Examine *don't know* very carefully. As Winston Churchill said, "Facts are better than dreams," and far better than nightmares. Take a stab at it; you'll gain confidence the more you practice.

I've left space at the end of this chapter. Take a few notes. Don't worry about defacing the book unless you've borrowed it from a library or a friend. The book police won't arrest you.

Also write down how you'd prefer or intend to feel. One of the things you're about to discover is that you have a lot of choices. For example, I never feel bad. I make a deliberate choice to feel good. I may have a cold or be tired, but I insist on my right to treat each new day as an opportunity for enjoyment and satisfaction.

Albert Einstein, the renowned physicist, said the most important life decision we make is deciding whether existence is essentially good or essentially bad.

More Than Likely Setting an Evolutionary Speed Record...

Conscious thought has almost entirely supplanted awareness as the prevailing operational state of the mind. Awareness still remains fully functional and functioning in the background, however. An emergency or emotional turmoil can bring awareness to the forefront: "I didn't think about it, I just rushed into the burning building." Otherwise, the thinking mind hijacks consciousness as a way to control events, either in the future (*prelive*) or the past (*relive*).

Freed from the domination of the thinking mind, the aware mind can keep you anchored in the moment encompassed by the "Now" as it receives and responds to the present's panoply of stimuli, which are charged with living, positive, high wavelength energy as opposed to attracting forms of energy that feature essentially negative properties—including entropic forces of obstruction and destruction—sought by the thinking mind. Awareness isn't passive; rather, it is a grateful acceptance of enlightenment generated by unfiltered and undistorted perceptions. I'll have more to say about negative energy as we go forward. For the moment, to get a taste of negative energy close your eyes and slowly, with emphasis, say aloud: "Failure, catastrophe, ruin, lies." Pause for a moment to let the meaning sink in. Notice your mood darkening. Negative energy is smothering your enthusiasm and hope.

What Do You Expect?

When I ask a new Egoscue Method client how she feels and get a shrug in reply, it tells me that I am dealing with a person who does not expect to feel good—and doesn't. How much of that feeling is self-inflicted by way of expectation? Plenty. Thoughts are things. They exist as energy, and as such they generate force, heat and momentum.

Frequently, a client will tell me about how much his back or knee hurts. I'll recommend a small postural adjustment. "How do you feel now?"

"It hurts."

"Really? Right now?"

"Well.... not right now. The pain has gone away. But it'll come back."

"So, the answer is your back doesn't hurt?"

"Yeah," they reluctantly admit, though in their mind expecting to be in pain amounted to the practical equivalent of actually being in pain.

And that brings us to the notorious "placebo effect." Several studies show that anywhere from thirty to fifty percent of the participants in certain experimental drug-testing programs experienced improvement in their medical conditions after receiving doses of inert pharmacological compounds (concocted from ingredients that were nothing more potent than sugar, simple starches and water, for instance) packaged and presented to resemble the real thing. Some skeptics dismiss the phenomenon as the scientific equivalent of UFO sightings—i.e., random outbreaks of localized collective lunacy. Others, including me, see what happened with placebos and continues to happen, as raising the possibility that just the anticipated benefits aroused by the comforting trappings of medical care from pill bottles to white coats, care versus despair, hopeful action instead of fearful inaction make a big difference—possibly a game-changer. The act of taking, receiving, or even just considering the (sham) drug as part of a seemingly legitimate treatment regimen could be powerful enough to improve the health of roughly a third to a half of those tested. Hence, expectation may amount to effectuation—a housekeeping process the brain uses to help organize experience and emotion, which seems to have no direct leverage compared to the potential unequivocal impact of swift-kick-in-the-chops chemical intervention—and so performs a major role in ameliorating health problems.

Flaws in testing methodology or other factors may be involved, yet results like these have been surfacing since first extensively reported in the mid-1950s. If your mind can persuade the body that an inert pill makes you feel better or causes uncomfortable side effects, and the scenario actually plays out as posited, then this far-more-dramatic possibility looms larger than ever: Belief itself may have many powerful medicinal properties.

Could it be that belief changes conditions within the body? Or are the studies all wrong? Fifty percent of all patients are faking illness? Faking recovery? Vast numbers of the sick and injured in the tests are just lucky? Just unlucky? If you expect pain in your forty-year-old knees when you take a Sunday run in the park or expect that a cloudy winter day will make you glum, a fifty-fifty chance that that outcome will conform to expectation strongly suggests that the disease model, the prevailing understanding of what cures and what kills, may be wrong.

I hesitate to say that the body believes. I'm not at all reluctant, however, to point out that the body perceives. And by perceiving belief, a state of mind is generated that can lead to a state of action capable of overcoming great obstacles.

Pain and Purpose

To merely say that the human body is an extremely sensitive organism understates the case. Our cells bristle with transmitters and receptors that scan our internal environment and the inputs we receive from external sources. Nothing goes undetected. Reaction is swift. If we set off only a few of those receptors and transmitters by telling ourselves to expect trouble, the body will mobilize defensive resources. Consequently, we feel like a fortress under siege: the gates are closed, rations scarce, the guns loaded and cocked. No wonder we don't feel good!

Fear intensifies physical pain. A typical fear-based response to pain is to hold your breath, which only increases stress by reducing the oxygen flow and adding to the anxiety. Another fear-based response is to limit your physical activity. "I don't climb stairs anymore," Leroy told me recently. Why not? I asked. "Stairs hurt my knees," he said. But stairs are a piece of cake compared to climbing trees, scrambling up mountains, dancing a jig, bowling and many other challenges the knees easily handle. I told Leroy that avoiding stairs will soon mean he'll be avoiding hills, minor inclines, stepping off

a curb or stepping into the shower. By restricting his movement he will reduce and eventually lose his ability to move.
And the pain will probably spread to his hips, lower back and
elsewhere as it dutifully warns Leroy about what he is doing to
himself.

Pain is not your enemy. It helps to regard pain as a natural
occurrence that serves an important service: notification that
the body finds a condition, a state or a stimulus to be detrimental, ranging from the mildly irritating to the harmful. Immediately rushing to take painkilling medicine without first
reflecting on what the pain is telling you is unwise. The pill or
potion may ease the pain temporarily (with side effects, because there are always side effects) but whatever it is that
caused the pain is still there, only now, drugged, you can't feel
it. Seek a cure, not just treatment. You have nothing to be
afraid of. Nothing.

Take a deep breath, lots of deep breaths, relax, and pay attention to your body.

Fear is an extreme form of expectation. Those who are
fearful expect that they are about to be hurt, overwhelmed, defeated. Most of what we expect to happen never does, yet we
suffer the ill effects of our imaginary expectations as if they had
actually come to pass. Stay in the moment: By relearning to be
aware of how you really feel, as opposed to how you expect to
feel, you allow the body to summon its full resources and to
generate accurate assessments of what's really happening that
can be processed and bounced back to your aware mind in the
form of self-confidence, pleasure and, amazingly enough, perfect health and peace of mind.

No one likes to think that they are regarded by others as
afraid or that they allow fear to impair their judgment and actions. *Coward* is a fighting word, as are its non-English equiva-
lents. But rather than slugging it out, you need to understand that

being afraid is part of being human. Fear is built into your emotional matrix, and in purest form serves an important purpose.

I'm not questioning your courage, or suggesting that it is better to let go and succumb to fear merely because it comes as standard equipment. On the contrary, fear is often a disease—a killer, the mother of all lethal infections—because it diverts energy away from maintaining healthy physiological processes. Every organ is drained of important resources and left terribly vulnerable.

Those "modern epidemics" that the sensation-loving news impresarios chatter about—diabetes, autism, fibromyalgia, obesity, autoimmune disorders and the like—are primarily consequences of putting the body through the enormous stress of preparing to confront danger: Blood vessels dilate to absorb more oxygen, fast-twitch muscle fibers are primed, blood pressure increases, the optic nerves rev up, and the kidneys and other vital organs slow down to conserve energy.

Blandly put, fear is an override mechanism that interrupts lesser emotions and routine processes in the interest of getting one human being out of harm's way before it is too late. I'm committing only a slight exaggeration when I say that fear is the hydrogen bomb of our emotions: a last resort, over-the-top, existential response to an existential threat that is ultimately deadly to aggressors and defenders alike. Instead of going to war once or twice a year as our early ancestors did to defeat an enemy threat against the village or when a tiger came prowling around the watering hole, we live in an era where the fear button is pushed again and again. Humankind now lives, sickens and dies with the consequences of the trivialization of fear.

Bleak? Although the answer is yes, there is a way out. When living in the moment, fear is relatively rare. Go take a walk on the beach; you'll see (feel) what I mean. The interlude restores the soul and repairs the body. By your not being present, dwelling instead in the bomb shelter of the imagination, rerunning the past (where *could haves*, *would haves*, *should/shouldn't haves*, and *might haves* grumble and growl) and rehearsing the future (where it is always personal, always about me and more, more, more), the footprints in the sand lead to ground zero. You may still be strolling along a glorious beach, but your head is on a harmful journey elsewhere.

Keep in mind that fear is a natural state, part of an emotional vocabulary. You are free to accept or reject what it offers. Having mostly lost its original context as protector of last resort, fear offers an illusory sense of control that is contradicted by the body every step of the way—if ... if you become present and aware. Fear is about escape and evasion. It wants you to lie low, slink and scurry. By regaining postural balance you can escape the emotional firestorm and rediscover peace of mind.

Fear is the best of emotions and the worst of emotions. We owe it a special place of honor. Without fear, human beings would probably be extinct. Even so, a compelling case can be made that fear has outlived its usefulness and is today mostly a menace.

Fear comes in two basic variations: Fear Classic and Fear Lite. Classic, the original ur-fear, is so retro, so ponderous, it is hardly a mere emotion at all; more a force of nature, like a lightening bolt. When Fear Classic strikes it overrides most other physiological functions, switching off cogitation and subordinating all things to one purpose: survival. In a flash, the sight, smell, growl or grunt, and even the harmonic vibrations of one of the great terrestrial predators like a grizzly bear or our close cousin, the mountain gorilla, launch us into freeze-fight-(or)-flight mode. No rational analysis takes place. There's a click and we go to the Fear Classic channel without further ado.

Fear Lite is a mutation of Fear Classic. It is compact, specialized and user-friendly: a Hammond organ compared to a Wurlitzer. Fear Lite plays a mean blues, creepy dark-night-of-the-living-dead dirges, funk, gansta rap and a host of other emotionally negative tunes that make us feel threatened, uneasy and troubled but not blasted into the realm of freeze-fight-(or)-flight.

Our original emotional repertoire consisted largely of joy, courage, confidence, curiosity and peace of mind. It expanded over a period of close to a million years, changing texture, timbre and color in response to the way we spontaneously interacted and continue to interact with our environment. Fear Lite started out as occasional riffs, a little night music, some humming in the background, and gradually became a nearly inescapable, mesmerizing soundtrack.

Fear Classic used the prospect of sudden and almost certain death, the *motivator extraordinaire*, to keep our earliest ancestors from being served as lunch before they had a chance to take over the world. At the time, creatures with big paws, big jaws and big appetites were fairly common. Freeze-fight-(or)-flight may not have happened every day; nevertheless, most prehistoric humans got to experience the thrill of utter terror on more than one occasion. It made quite an impression. The echo of that terror resonated to such a degree and lingered in the memory bank that humans were able tone it down and use the diluted recollection to scare themselves into learning more routine life lessons: *If you put your hand in the fire again, sonny boy, it is going to hurt*, for instance. *Pick on somebody your own size next time*; *walk softly and carry a big stick.* By repeating these admonishments out loud, you may be able to detect a slight frisson of fear taking place in the borderlands of your conscious/unconscious mind that underscores the importance of the messages.

Through natural selection, Fear Lite was established as a teaching tool and became a mainstay of the thinking mind to the point that most contemporary men and women have almost forgotten how to reason without turning up the volume of the negative soundtrack: *My boss hates me, so I better not be late for work; Fred is going to stab me in the back, so I'll get him first; going to the gym is a drag, but if I don't I'll have a heart attack; I can't do this myself, I am not enough.*

The bad news is that most of us are awash in negative emotions. The good news is we can switch off the Fear Lite soundtrack and listen instead to the original emotional music: joy, courage, confidence, curiosity and peace of mind. And should a grizzly bear wander into your backyard, Fear Classic is still there to offer freeze-fight-(or)-flight. The second-best defense is a good defense.

From a practical standpoint, though, playing defense is cumbersome; you have to dig in and heavy up. However, fear is portable, available when needed, tucked away within reach when it's not. A quick squirt of Fear Classic cranks up the body to high alert.

Fortunately, the grizzly or wolf is not always at the door. In the roughest neighborhoods there were (and are) moments, hours, days or weeks of relative tranquility. When things calm down, fear backs off; all the freeze-fight-(or)-flight physiological changes quickly return to normal. The brain keeps a close watch to detect high levels of cortisol, a powerful stress hormone, and signals the adrenal gland to cut back on production as the danger passes.

This on-off switch allows for brief, highly stressful jolts of neural chemicals and hormones which, if prolonged, damage the internal systems. Wisely, there is no fixed cutoff point that would disable the fear mechanism after a set period of activation because it is impossible to know how frequently predator and prey will come into contact. The body wants a fear cocktail on hand just in case there's a sudden plague of crocodiles. It is a tradeoff of risking possibly harmful short-term stress balanced against a truly long-term proposition—death.

These days the big predators are much fewer in number, which should mean that for most of us the fear switch can remain off. Alas, that's not the case.

Fear—the worst of emotions—is as much a ubiquitous feature of the modern era as the cell phone. To put the body into freeze-fight-(or)-flight mode, the perception of danger must cross a far higher emotional threshold than one that would occur in the case of an argument with a neighbor or a confrontation with an enemy from another tribe. For a healthy, balanced, fully functional person, such lower-intensity situations can be handled without the need to hit the panic button.

The balanced body's internal monitors are fully aware of the available inner resources—strength, stamina, speed, ingenuity and, most of all, energy. It regards the existing conditions and environment, as perceived by the senses and by the body's multitude of sophisticated scanners, to be entirely within the individual's power to cope. There may be minor physiological adjustments but nothing like Fear Classic, the *run-hide-fight-for-your-life* response triggered by a large predator. But when balance is disrupted, such a nuanced reading cannot take place. Much of the firepower of Fear Classic activates by default because the body must guess whether it has the physical capabilities to survive. It assumes the worst and acts accordingly.

Today, postural imbalance has left many people bereft of resources—energy reserves are so skimpy that relatively minor challenges trigger bio-chemical and physiological weaponry associated with the freeze-fight-(or)-flight response. Called on to assess danger, the body reads that preexisting lack of energy as incontrovertible evidence that it doesn't have the resources to survive without blasting the system into overdrive. At the same time, Fear Lite, with its negative emotional beat, is pounding away, intensifying the sense of fear and danger. Consequently, minor conflicts, frustrations, and surprises trigger physiological responses worthy of wrestling a python. For many people the rumble in the jungle is nonstop.

In theory, anything as destructive as fear should have long ago goaded the body into devising a way to keep freeze-fight-(or)-flight responses safely locked in a cage and released only in the event of maximum danger. Since it lacks hardly any energy reserves, fear is so stimulating that it is addictive. Modern men and women get high on fear, both Classic and Lite. Drained of energy, their bodies use fear to kick-start their physiological systems, to rev them up, which further exacerbates the energy brown-out and leaves them dependent on using a powerful, last-resort stimulant as a matter of routine.

Not only does constant fear cause constant severe physiological stress, it burns through an already dwindling energy supply to handle even the most run-of-the-mill events. The immune system, which requires abundant energy, is compromised and the body soon loses it ability to fight off physical and mental illness, aging and accidental injuries.

Fear is particularly dangerous because it locks you out of the present moment and blocks the awareness you need to be in contact with your body. What with the clanging of neural, chemical and hormonal warnings, little else gets through. The fear message—with its context of dangerously inadequate resources—prompts you to turn outside of yourself for help. Getting control and keeping control of your health (even if it means giving that control to others) is a fear-based strategy; the body's sensitive stimulus-and-response mechanism requires you to be an empathetic observer—not an exacting, fiat-issuing controller.

One of the biggest problems facing health care providers is breaking through the wall of fear that seals off individuals from the help they desperately need. Fear freezes many people in place. The awareness necessary to keep them attuned to what the body needs is drowned out. Change becomes impossible. Instead, to preserve the status quo–and conserve what little energy remains–people seek drastic remedies that would otherwise be shunned. They turn away from an internal response supported by a knowing peace of mind toward an unsupported, fear-based, external response.

Fear is the dominant emotion of the modern age. It destroys peace of mind and harms your health. By ratcheting down the level of fear and ratcheting up high wavelength energy through restoring a balanced posture–you can see it and feel it happen–it is possible to give the body's internal wisdom and strength a chance to be heard and a chance to prevail.

Please stand up. It won't take long; this is a quickie. Close your eyes (after reading these instructions, of course), take a deep breath, but stand without deliberately balancing your weight and aligning your musculoskeletal system they way you did in Chapter 2. All set? Now say the words "It is broken" aloud three times. Pause, take another deep breath and say "Peace of mind" three times.

Did you notice a difference? Many people do, and some don't. So try it again.

For those who do feel a difference, the first part of the exercise tends to produce low-level tension, an up-tick of anxiety. The second part produces a feeling of calmness with a distinct awareness of inner peace. By standing in an unbalanced position, you did not draw extra high wavelength energy from the universal power grid. Instead,

> **Going Deeper**
>
> *Power vs. Force* by Dr. David R. Hawkins and published by Hay House is a valuable introduction to the concept of positive and negative energy. It is not a 'quick read' or a 'page-turner,' but it is well worth the effort.

> **Aligning Actions with Ideas**
> *You must live your ideas. It doesn't upgrade your energy quality if you think "giving" and act "taking."*

you reacted to the energy content of the words you said aloud. If you were muscle-tested, a standard albeit controversial technique of kinesiology, there would likely be a measurable decrease in muscle strength when you repeated the words "It is broken." In general this is typical of negative words, stressful emotional states and even substances such as toxic drugs, sugar, salt and many other things we have subconsciously learned are better to avoid. The muscles are ex-pressing that awareness by weakening or strengthening slightly as they react to the energy levels generated when a person holds the substance or, as in this example, when they say the words aloud (words are things, and things are energy).

David R. Hawkins, M.D., Ph.D., a pioneering author and researcher, has compiled an extensive glossary of positive words paired with their negative counterparts, which he has cross-tested and ranked numerically according to their "At-tractor energy" patterns. Saying the words aloud or just read-ing them silently produces a measurable response. The higher the number, the more beneficial the effect. Lower numbers correlate with lower-frequency energy waves, which are a sim-pler, extremely basic form of energy that blocks the receiver from taking in higher-frequency energy that delivers far more power.

When you lose musculoskeletal system balance and suc-cumb to fear, your thinking mind is awash in negative words and ideas that create a sort of set point or incoming channel that attracts only low wavelength energy to your body. Hawkins has demonstrated that like attracts like; there's no room left for high wavelength energy. You end up with a think-ing mind crammed full of inferior-grade energy that can't pos-sibly keep your health from deteriorating and, in fact, directly contributes to its decline, which is why it is referred to as "Sub-tractor energy" or "Subtractive energy." It explains why self-destructive acts form bad habits and are often repeated: Sub-tractive energy can't support your better angels. The drunk has only enough lower wavelength energy to pour another drink; the liar cannot tell the truth because he doesn't have enough Attractor energy to beat back the easy falsehood.

Hawkins believes that you can upgrade your energy qual-ity by consciously choosing positive, life-affirming ideas and actions—for instance, "giving" draws superior incoming high wavelength energy that lifts the human spirit, whereas "taking" does not—and I agree. But it is a difficult word-by-word uphill climb that is ultimately doomed to failure unless you restore musculoskeletal system balance and reestablish a full high wavelength energy connection to the universal power grid.

As you discovered doing the simple exercise in this chap-ter, it's possible to get a small up-tick in peace of mind simply by changing the words you say aloud (or think silently) from negative to positive. However, it is a small trickle of high-quality energy.

You can do a lot better than that. Go ahead, change fear-based words and ideas—and change your posture by restoring balance.

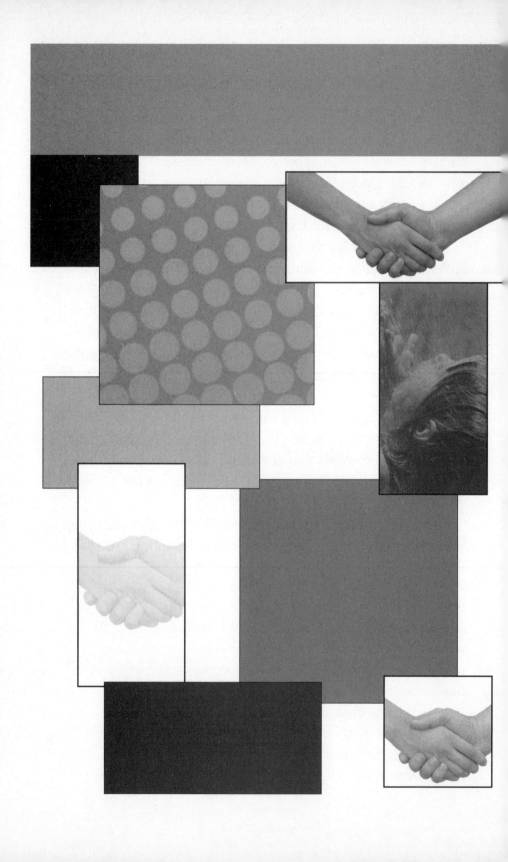

Muscle Magic

The brain is, well, brainy; the reproductive organs sexy; and the thumb very useful for hitch-hiking and tool-making, but I am not persuaded that humans owe our special *alpha-mammal* status to anything other than the musculoskeletal system.

Mere muscle and bone, connecting tissue, jointure, and a gossamer neural tapestry put you into an upright position, balanced on two feet, and allow you to walk, run, turn to the left and right, spin around, reach out and up, use your hands to throw baseballs and snowballs, make love, pray, write sonnets, wage war and sign peace treaties. I could go on and on. In terms of sheer variety, the human locomotion repertoire is indeed extraordinary.

And yet unlike our other major physiological arrangements, the musculoskeletal system gives the impression (a misimpression, for sure) of being rather haphazard, even crude in function and form–

too many moving parts, flat spots and low-tech compromises. To most students of human anatomy, one small intestine is pretty much like any other small intestine. The same goes for healthy lungs and hearts: more or less the same coherent package from person to person; a collection of conduits, bellows, filters and pumps. However, the musculoskeletal system comes in a variety of homely shapes and sizes—and not because of sloppy quality control or crude design. I can offer at least two good reasons. One, it operates in a far more eclectic external environment than any other physiological system and, two, the musculoskeletal system provides the means of locomotion for individuals who differ widely in weight, height, muscular strength, stamina, habits and activity levels.

Arguably, the musculoskeletal system has far more direct external interaction than other internal systems, which are tucked away deep inside the body's protective envelope; your left ventricle doesn't stub its valves on rocks or bang up its knees playing basketball. Only skin has more exposure to earth, water, wind and fire—let alone suffer insect bites, poison ivy, and razor burn. Our world is a rough place of many extremes; the sheer number of plausible ways to live, work and play in it is huge. While the skin and other organs go along for the ride, the musculoskeletal system is the ride. We move it, and it moves us until we die.

Consequently, there is a wide range of performance—and that can be misleading: Mary is tall and thin, walks

---

Muscle – Part 1

Muscles have two major functions: They contract (the fibers shorten) and relax (the fibers lengthen). No other tissue in the body does this. The result is motion, an ability to accomplish an immense number and variety of tasks, activities and acrobatics.

Skeletal muscles move bones because they are attached to bones at both ends of a muscle via tendons. The origin tendon at one end of the muscle is closest to the spinal axis, and the "insertion" tendon is farther from the axis. By shortening its fibers, a muscle draws the bone near the insertion toward the anchor and the body's spinal axis.

with a slight limp on the right side, and is an okay winter weekend ice skater, but tires easily; Joe, short and fat, can't swivel his head more than a few degrees in either direction, spends much of his day at a desk or sitting in front of the TV at night, and has insomnia. Meanwhile, Sharon, an Olympic athlete, breaks records using the exact same musculoskeletal equipment (the same, that is, in terms of design function). For both Mary and Joe, the cumulative lifetime performance of their musculoskeletal systems, measured by miles traveled, loads lifted, and the daily dance routine of stretching, bending, twisting, turning and artfully using their hands, is actually a remarkable display of endurance and physical prowess, although it falls far short of the full potential approached by Sharon or other star athletes. Such wide disparity is typical—most people are more like Mary and Joe than Sharon—and it contributes to the notion that the musculoskeletal system is, in general, an inferior piece of work: frail, accident-prone, and inconsistent.

Aspiring anatomical architects and engineers fancy that they can devise a better spine, a stronger knee, a longer-lasting hip. Maybe it is an utter lack of imagination on my part, but when I look at Mary or Joe I see a truly ingenious solution to a nearly intractable problem—giving reliable structure and coherent, multi-directional movement to 206 or so skeletal

> **More Muscle – Part 2**
>
> To move the bone back to the starting point, the contracting muscle relaxes to allow the fibers to lengthen but does not actually push or pull. Instead, a second opposing muscle, part of a working pair, contracts to accomplish the return trip.
>
> By working in pairs, muscles alternate contracting-relaxing and relaxing-contracting to allow the body, for example, to bend over and then stand up straight. But if one muscle contracts only partially or doesn't fully relax, the bones cannot return to a completely vertical position. The body does allow for temporary variations in contraction-relaxation to account for different situations. But over time, the body "forgets" and loses access to its fully functional alignment and balance.

> **Just in Case**
>
> As I explained in my book *Pain Free*, the design of the musculoskeletal system allows for temporary misalignment in case of accidents or unusual, life-or-death conditions when the system is under stress, but only for a short time. Many people subject themselves to a nearly permanent state of misalignment lasting for years. Something has to give, and it does.

bones without falling, crawling, hopping, slithering or flapping. Just being able to stand up, bear our own weight and remain in place is a remarkable achievement. Walking is a miracle of coordination! No matter how it happened, we are lucky that our ancestors got an apparatus that allowed them and us to counteract gravity, to stand upright on two feet, and to smoothly walk and run from point A to point B—because we'd never be able to invent it from scratch on our own. Today's prosthetic devices are rough approximations of the original limbs they replace; far from perfect despite all of our self-proclaimed technological savvy.

When there is pain, limitation or other problems, the design and quality of the musculoskeletal system aren't at fault as much as the way we are using and misusing the design and its component parts. Our upright, balanced, bipedal posture is a product of the messy, improvisatory business of climbing down from the trees, getting the head up over the tall grass, the eyes wide open, and the forepaws off the ground so they could hold a weapon, tools and extra food supplies. Until that occurred, our distant ancestors were a bunch of hapless primates, the favorite lunchmeat of carnivores no bigger than French poodles. For reasons we can only guess at, humankind stood up, started moving and rarely stopped.

Going vertical required skeletal alignment, flexible and resilient jointure, close muscular coordination and orchestration, and a means of staying upright. Voilà! A two-legged, anti-gravity machine, an all-weather, all-terrain SUV emerged from the mist of time. It is obvious that simple skeletal misalignment drastically impedes the paramount function of the musculoskeletal system. Today, millions of Marys and Joes are slowly collapsing out of vertical alignment, losing their battle with gravity, thanks to a sedentary modern lifestyle. They don't even get the minimal levels of motion required to maintain adequate muscle strength and engagement to support spinal function, skeletal alignment, balance, and proper joint interaction and articulation.

The Egoscue Method was devised to restore alignment by reintroducing motion that strengthens and re-engages temporarily dysfunctional supporting muscles and other musculoskeletal components. I call it *postural therapy*, a way to address injury and chronic pain without resorting to toxic drugs or invasive surgical procedures; also, it is an effective technique for achieving peak athletic conditioning.

Or so I thought. Actually, I was right but had the wrong reason. I blundered when I looked at the evidence and concluded that postural therapy is effective because skeletal misalignment is bad, and proper alignment is good. From a literal and superficial standpoint, that's true. It begs the question, however.

Why?

Here's where we circle back to the exercise I asked you to do in Chapter 2. The primary purpose of the musculoskeletal system—*numero uno*—is to download and circulate high wavelength energy to fuel the sixty trillion cells in the typical adult body. Musculoskeletal system misalignment, visible and measurable, is a reliable indicator of the body's lack of capacity to take on energy supplies. Hence, postural alignment—balance—is both cause and effect: All the body's internal systems function more powerfully because adequate energy resources are available, and in turn that enhanced function leads to the uptake of more energy, more capacity, and an increasingly healthy life. While the musculoskeletal system moves us, it also fuels us.

What's more, a strong, properly aligned and engaged musculoskeletal system makes it possible for your body's internal sensory apparatus to precisely monitor and choreograph the complex interplay of the chemical, electrical, biomechanical and cellular processes. Simply by standing up on two feet—an overt act not unlike the act of tuning an antenna—the body is informed within fractions of seconds how well the liver is functioning and whether the heart is straining. Messages by the billions streak up the spine to the brain, and orders race back down: Sample, adjust, tweak, recalibrate, sample again.... A misaligned musculoskeletal system triggers a host of warnings that activate hormonal responses that affect your mood, respiration, blood pressure, energy levels and resistance to illness.

Not only does misalignment interfere with the flow of message traffic, it sends messages of its own announcing that the body is literally losing its life. Stiffness and immobility are two characteristics of a corpse. By cutting off oxygen, freezing joints and contracting muscles, the musculoskeletal system concedes that gravity is winning, must win. Every *this* yields every *thus*: Human sacrifice takes place. The flesh, bone and blood capsule becomes inert while the spirit cuts loose from the wreckage to be repurified as nothing more or less than positive energy.

Now I'm going to get a little technical—just a little. It is as if we have two metabolic loops, one for processing and utilizing energy derived from eatable protein and carbohydrate matter, and another for ingesting and digesting high wavelength energy that radiates through the space we inhabit. Without the high wavelength energy loop, the carbo/protein metabolic loop is under siege, struggling to keep the various internal systems efficient and healthy, but losing ground over time. By firing up both loops simultaneously there is plenty of energy. The musculoskeletal system not only provides routine locomotion, it supplies this additional power to the entire body in sufficient quantities to mean the difference between a spotty subsistence existence and today's vast global human civilization; and, just in case we are too busy or too unaware to pay attention, it tells us directly, unmistakably, whether our energy intake is high or low.

Your car has a fuel gauge even though it will be obvious—and inconvenient—when the tank runs dry. The human body has one as well. Instead of a little arrow pointing at ½, your shoulders and spine do the pointing by rounding and slumping; you lose skeletal alignment, and with it, balance is also lost. As the head begins to hang forward and down (and other musculoskeletal components lose their verticality), the *arrow* goes to ¼ or less. As a result, major posture muscles are losing even more of their energy charge; tone, length and strength are dwindling.

The musculoskeletal system plainly displays, in real time, how much or how little energy is aboard. I suspect that our earliest ancestors chose mates, hunting partners, and leaders by intuitively making alliances with those who *looked right*. They read the body language, the posture, and correlated it to the likelihood of success based on the appearance of those who had succeeded in the past. An upright, balanced posture was empirical evidence of strength, stamina and prehistoric street smarts.

Today, your posture is capable of sending the same positive message or delivering a dire warning. At issue—and it's a biggie—is whether you are capable of being aware of those messages. I believe you are; you've got all the right equipment, and that is why I'm going to keep yammering at you about the importance of musculoskeletal balance.

Balance, balance and more balance…. You either have it or you are losing your perfect health.

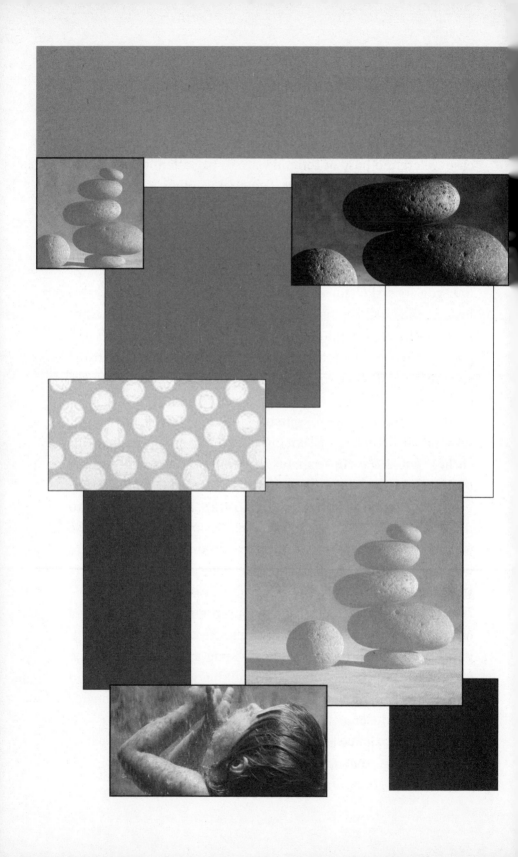

Balance of Forces

From the very first days of human history, success and failure, perfect health and serious illness, happiness and despair have had distinct postures. We wear our health like a cloak.

Just as a modern sailor knows how to interpret subtle changes in wind direction, currents and cloud cover to predict weather patterns (they'll tell you they can *feel* that the weather is about to change), Neolithic warrior chiefs and Ancient Roman generals could forecast the impending victory or defeat of their armies by watching the way the infantry marched into battle.

Those commanders carefully inspected their troops—noted an uncertain gait, restricted arm swing, labored pace—and accurately foresaw disaster ahead. Or more auspicious reviews discerned heads held high, squared shoulders, self-confidence, boundless energy and fierce joy that presaged triumph. Pure *wysiwyg* (what you see is what you get). Yet those leaders would probably have scoffed at the idea that they could read the army's combined musculoskeletal arsenal the same way they could inspect and evaluate a battery of catapults or a squadron of cavalry. Rather it was a regarded as a hunch, intuition, a gut check, maybe even magic. Actually, it was more than mere magic: They were tapping into a special human resource—feelings drawn from a deep pool of emotions linked to an even deeper reservoir of collective experience.

The solitary soldier felt it too and also knew the meaning.

Today, the posture you see continues to be what you get—and what you feel. But many of us have been persuaded to distrust and ignore the feelings conveyed by our posture. Instead of listening to those messengers and taking heed, we try to silence them with powerful drugs, invasive medical procedures and the opinions of others; a huge irony since many of us are certainly descendents of men and women who were acutely aware of their own feelings, acted on them and lived to fight another day (and pass on their genes).

Did they at least suspect that what they saw and felt was the result of musculoskeletal system balance or the lack of it? I doubt it. The body informs, it doesn't explain. Explanations are the work of the thinking mind, a far less reliable process of the brain than is the aware mind, which deals in feelings—e.g., does this stimulus feel good or bad? Is it enjoyable or not? They used their aware mind to choose the ways and means to sustain positive feelings that were being generated or, if the feelings were negative, to avoid as best they could whatever it was that was producing bad feelings. The truth doesn't need an explanation or expert validation; instead, it must feel right.

Never Mind

Have you lost your mind? Don't bother looking under the chair.
You never had one. The brain actually exists as corporal matter.
A surgeon can open the skull of a living human and examine
brain tissue. There is no mind, however. It's been described—ludi-
crously, I believe—as an immaterial substance. A what? The mind
is more usefully understood as a process of the brain for recording
and organizing experience. The mind is in effect a faulty memory.
Faulty because it leaks its contents—memories, lingering displace-
ment patterns of energy waves associated with past events—into
our consciousness instead of keeping them sealed away in the
background.

The memory, as repository of non-extant stimulus, seems to be
walled off from the present in other creatures; nonetheless, it informs
and helps shape present actions. For instance, a hungry seagull learns
that hanging out at the town dump is a way to get food, but the bird
doesn't consciously think about the connection, much less deliberately assign value. The stomach rumbles and wings flap to the nearest
landfill. The scruffy gourmand learns to repeat a past action over and
over again, but doesn't reason. That last step—reasoning—happens
only to creatures with leaky memories who have reasoned themselves
into possession of a mind and spent the better part of a hundred
thousand years developing that faculty by reliving the past and trying
to control the future.

Indeed, *what you see is what you get* is true. And *what you
feel is what you get* is even truer. Posture is the mechanism
that guides human beings to this essential fact. Balance feels
good, imbalance feels bad. Without balance you cannot access
your aware mind; all emotions except fear are walled off, out
of reach. But full-blown fear was relatively uncommon (see
Chapter 4). Pleasure was a more familiar emotion, as was its
linkage to success and self-confidence.

The human body is extremely sensitive to imbalance because it can only be caused by lack of adequate high wavelength energy. They didn't know high wavelength energy from

Zeus' thunderbolts, but when those marching Roman legion-
naires were balanced, they consequently felt invincible. They
had the inner resources—strength, stamina and willpower—to
conquer the world. Out of balance, they felt vulnerable, and
they were.

By rediscovering the primary purpose of musculoskeletal
system balance and achieving that balance, you are in a position to reclaim an important health legacy:

Peace of mind.

Hold on; don't write off peace of mind as a hippy-dippy,
space cadet state of goofy detachment. Peace of mind is the
pillar that supports courage, wisdom and happiness.

The exercise that you did in Chapter 2 demonstrates that
peace of mind awaits your summons. When you plug into the
universal power grid by balancing your posture and drawing
on its high wavelength energy, the mental and physical static
quiets down; in its place are clarity and focus. The incoming
energy flow smoothes the turbulence by augmenting and supporting the metabolic power required to renew the body's
cells, fuel them, and build, maintain and operate your many
systems. This infusion of high wavelength energy serves to remove waste, fight disease and allow you, in general, to kick
back and enjoy life's pleasures. You are able to live in the
present where the aware mind connects to feelings that accurately convey what the body needs to remain optimally
healthy.

The small taste of that was what you experienced in Chapter 2 by briefly getting your posture into a rough semblance of
balance:

• Your weight was equally balanced on both feet side-to-side
  and front-to-back

• Your load-bearing joints (ankles, knees, shoulders and hips)
  were vertically aligned

- Those joints, arranged in pairs, were also aligned horizontally on parallel planar surfaces side-to-side
- There was an S-curve in the spine that held the upper torso upright
- Shoulders were back over the hips and aligned as a pair on each side
- The head was level, riding on your neck (the top of the spine) in vertical alignment over the pelvis
- Imaginary lines drawn through these musculoskeletal components formed 90-degree angles and a stable but flexible, ladder-like structure

If someone had snapped a picture of you at the time you were doing the exercise, you would have seemed younger, stronger, healthier, and happier.

All About Balance

Postural balance looks good—because it is good. We like the look of it because we value the feel of it even more. Far more than comeliness or athletic talent that some people have and others lack, balance perfectly equips each individual to move freely while at the same time guarding his or her own health. Balance is not optional. Without balance, those who believe the human body cannot cope with the demands of modern life are correct. There is no substitute for postural balance.

One look at our friends Mary and Joe from Chapter 5 tells me all I need to know—they are out of balance and, consequently, badly lack energy. Their postures do not reflect age, accidents, heredity, disease or bad habits. Diet, weekly trips to the gym, joint replacement or exotic pharmaceutical concoctions won't offer much lasting help. The best remedy for what ails Mary and Joe is the courage to make their own decisions based on how they *feel* about their health. Courage requires energy–a lot of energy. By returning to postural balance, they'll top off their depleted energy supplies, obtain the inner resources to make corrective changes, and put an end to years of being unaware of the important things their bodies have been trying to tell them. They'll have peace of mind. And in the event that those "important things" include warnings of serious illness brought on by their long-term energy deficits–which the body is hard-wired to detect–Mary and Joe will be aware of them and aware of what has to be done.

By returning to musculoskeletal system balance, they can access the flow of limitless energy that brings peace of mind, lack of fear, and strength to heal. Without balance, all of us are left in double jeopardy: We lack enough high wavelength energy to sustain our health, and lack the assurance–let's hear it for national health assurance–that our emotions give us as reliable feedback on whether our actions (lifestyle, choices, habits, etc.) are helping or hurting. Humans have a subtle yet immensely powerful emotional apparatus assigned to perform those missions; to be cut off from it is a sad fate for creatures that have clocked more than a million years by relying on the emotional *feel* of things rather than the *think* of things (to borrow a phrase attributed to Stanley Kubrick, the great film director).

I do not see it as a choice between modern medical care and faith-healing. Yes, faith is involved–faith in yourself, faith in your innate ability to act in your own best interest. Yet faith does not preclude using technology or expertise as long as your emotional radar is switched on. As complicated as medical treatment has become, you can still keep faith with the body's unerring wisdom, but only if you regain and maintain balance.

   Still have doubts about the essential role of postural balance? I'm not surprised. Don't take my word for it—words rely too heavily on the think of things. Get the feel of it for yourself and then you'll be ready to live well, and do it with peace of mind.

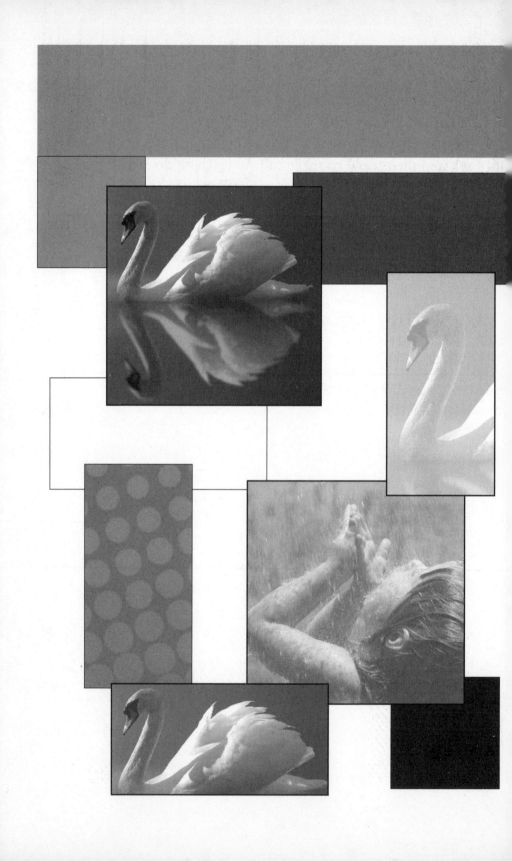

Halo ... Halo ...

I would like to introduce you to another feeling. This one is generated by an exercise similar to the one I asked you to do in Chapter 2, only it is a little more dramatic. I am assuming—and believe me, it is a safe assumption—that you are way out of balance and running low on positive, high wavelength energy. If not, good on you, as my Aussie friends say; a brief refresher course won't hurt at all. The demonstration of Attractor energy can be underwhelming to some people because their energy resources are so depleted that the small spurt of energy that is generated by using positive words as opposed to negative words can be difficult for them to detect.

With this exercise, you can raise the intensity of the feeling and at the same time produce a sensation that for most people is unambiguously beneficial. In other words, I think you're going to like it.

Stand naturally; e.g., like you normally do. Don't square up or try to balance yourself. Similar to the exercise last time, I want you to be initially in an unbalanced state. Okay, look around the room you are in. Spot something that you don't like. A crooked picture frame, a pile of newspapers, a cluttered shelf. There is usually something out there that's less than perfect. Your thinking mind is a critic; you'll find something not to like.

Stare at the mess, let it sink in. Tune in to how it makes you feel—anger at yourself for not cleaning up; exasperated; determined to fix things; surprised. One Egoscue Clinic client did this exercise over the phone from his office and experienced a slight feeling of breathlessness when he noticed his supply closet was a slum. He was ashamed. You should definitely have a reaction to what seems like confirmation that you are not in complete control of your environment.

Close your eyes for about a minute and then open again. And there is the same mess across the room; it hasn't moved.

Now close your eyes and square up: head, neck and shoulders back, feet hips-width apart, weight balanced evenly on the balls of each foot. Take a few deep breaths and exhale. Stay there for about a minute and then open your eyes.

Behold the trouble spot. What does it feel like now? Focus. Give it a moment. Has that original reaction from the unbalanced position changed? Is there new information reaching you?

Many people immediately sense that the mess, the trouble spot, has become far less important. The urgency is gone, the pressure off. The flaking paint on the ceiling can wait ... the supply closet is fine. They are getting a flow of high wavelength energy that is telling them, "This is no big deal. Relax."

Let's try something else. Sit down, take a short break. I want you to lapse back into an unbalanced state. Stand up, keep your posture natural. No cheating; you don't usually stand with your shoulders pulled back like that. Let them roll forward.

Everyone has a sense of their personal space. Can you estimate yours? Where does your personal space, that small zone that you prefer to keep open and clear of intruders, begin? One foot out? Two or three? When a stranger approaches too closely and you become uncomfortable, he has invaded your personal space.

Estimate the size of that zone and close your eyes. Go through all the squaring and balancing up procedures we used earlier. Don't forget your feet–parallel, and straight ahead, hips-width apart, balance the weight equally side to side and front to back. Hold the posture for two minutes.

Open your eyes. How far out does the personal space extend now?

Yeah, it's increased, perhaps by three or four feet.

You have an aura, an energy field that radiates out from your body much like the halos on saints depicted by 14th-century Italian painters. Perhaps Saint Francis of Assisi actually walked around with his hair on fire, but I tend to doubt it. More likely, artists could feel the saint's energy and were moved to give it a concrete expression in the form of a halo.

As you lose balance and energy, your aura shrinks. There's certainly not enough to light up a halo, and personal space no longer demarks a zone under your control but one that has been breached and cannot supply a sense of security. A "distant," "cold," and "guarded" person is struggling to protect herself from the loss of her aura by throwing up a wide defensive perimeter. Before, she became anxious when people came within a foot or two. Now, as her aura drains away, being in the same room with a stranger is troubling. The overriding impulse is to run and hide.

A Closer Look at Auras and Comfort Zones

For the purposes of our discussion, let's define energy as the capacity for action. The human body is a highly organized system with a truly impressive capacity and wide range for taking action in at least three forms: as rote repetitive action, as innovative first-of-its-kind action that arises in response to a new experience, and as involuntary action without conscious volition, like a heartbeat. In other words, to address the first and second of the three categories, we can remember how we moved an hour ago and duplicate that action if need be, or we act in new and different ways without prior experience or pre-programming. The important point is that sudden, unexpected changes in circumstances that require innovative action are not major challenges. Witness human history and the unprecedented actions recorded in everything from arts to sports. Our innovative action adeptness generates a distinct attitude or mood that has come to be known as an optimistic outlook. Through a working partnership of 1) the physical functions that directly carry out innovative acts, and 2) the mind that accepts the innovative requirement emotionally while supporting it cognitively, this optimism leads us to intuitively understand and embrace change as a beneficial process.

Optimism seeks the long view; it regards the unavoidable events of life–pain, rejection, disappointments–not as insurmountable obstacles or distressing symptoms to be treated in crisis mode but as part of the natural process of change. "Taking things in stride" is an optimistic life view. This attitude exists only as long as the individual retains full capacity for action; i.e., absolute emotional certainty that he has the inner resources to successfully manage change without fear of failure.

The challenge with this, of course, is the lower the external energy frequency the less capable we become moment to moment, day to day, week to week. Pessimism replaces optimism.

There is no pill you can take to restore a lost aura, although many medications attempt to simulate a response that superficially resembles a charged-up energy field–sleeplessness, high blood pressure, rapid heartbeat, jumpiness, impulsive behavior

(or its polar opposite, indecision) and the like. Medical re-
searchers keep looking for ways to replace the "broken" part
that produces the aura or other "lost" physiological functions.
Broken?
Lost?
Not!

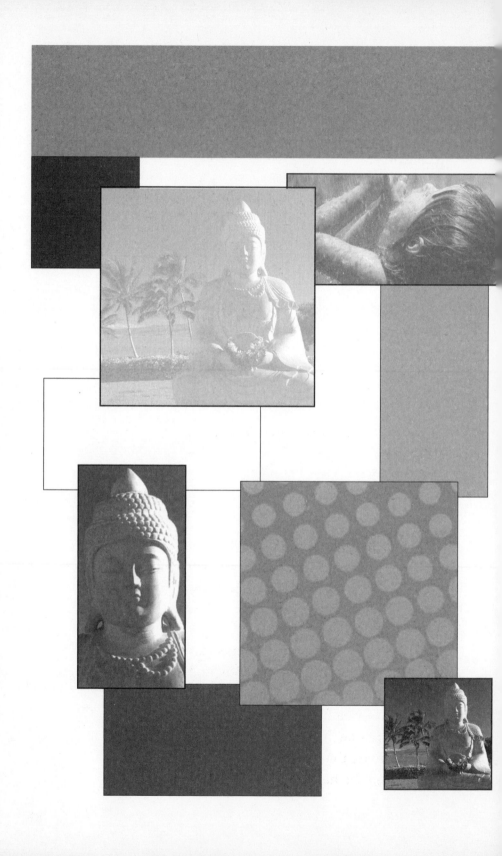

Storytellers

*"Sing to me of the man, Muse, the man of twists
and turns ..."*

As one who stands in awe of the human musculoskeletal system with its splendid carrying capacity
for heroism and folly, rereading Robert Fagles'
translation of the first line of the *Odyssey* always
stuns me.

Before pausing for breath, Homer casts a magic
spell to conjure up a "man of twists and turns ...,"
deftly capturing our legacy of muscle and movement
to drag it forth in a net of words that sing with rest-
less echoes of the fateful consequences of actions
taken, "... driven time and again off course, once he
had plundered the hallowed heights of Troy."

Many cities of men he saw and learned their minds,
Many pains he suffered, heartsick on the open sea,
Fighting to save his life and bring his comrades home.
But he could not save them from disaster, hard as he strove—
The recklessness of their own ways destroyed them all,
the blind fools, they devoured the cattle of the Sun
and the Sungod blotted out the day of their return.
Launch out on his story, Muse, daughter of Zeus,
start from where you will—sing for our time too.

Storytelling is the theme of this chapter and one of the most important elements of the book you are now reading. Odysseus—the man of twists and turns—is the first Everyman of literature, not counting Enkidu, a character in the 4000-year-old *Epic of Gilgamesh*, carved on stone tablets, buried in an Mesopotamian desert and discovered a century ago. Enkidu has his fans, yet as a proxy or double for the Babylonian warrior god Gilgamesh, he rode on supernatural coattails—not fair!—and therefore loses stature.

Fiction, whether it is epic verse or modern potboilers, is a form of biography, an account of events and adventures that take place as the quest for life's meaning unfolds. Odysseus and Enkidu discover that nothing is permanent, everything changes—and keeps changing.

The realization came as a great shock to fictional characters and real people. Modern storytellers still grapple with the implications. All living things are in permanent negotiations with their environment over what must be done to accommodate change.

Each of us creates a story that explains who we are and why we are. Like Homer, we commit it to memory (not paper, not even granite tablets) and thereby imbue the story with transcendent power. Shakespeare's *Hamlet* begins with the question that launches all stories: "Who's there?" Nearly four hours later the suspects have been rounded up—adulterers, murderers, lunatics, the heartbroken, vengeance-seekers, the unlucky, and all the rest is silence.

Without exception, visitors to an Egoscue Method clinic bring a story with them. I suspect that is also true for every other alternative and mainstream health care operation in the world. People never leave home without their story.

Over the years, I have learned to listen closely to those stories and I have discovered just how important they are. The narratives can be filled with insightful information, plot points, character development, surprises, growth, confusion, crisis and suspense. Many physicians (and other health practitioners) think they don't have time for these stories. They speed-listen for ten minutes, home in on the usual symptomatic suspects, order up a few tests and diagnose. Newtonian micro-medicine—the quest to find the broken part, no matter how small—rules out other options. *Gotta keep digging deeper! Fix what's broken! Move on!*

In the process, there is a huge disconnect. The physician is unable to make more than a cursory use of an invaluable resource, and the patient cannot determine whether the person he or she has turned to for help fully understands their situation. The uncertainty can cast a dark shadow over the relationship at the precise moment it needs to be on the firmest possible footing.

So, it is another example of bad doctors and good patients who are poorly served, right? No, not really.

The fault lies with the stories. Severe musculoskeletal system imbalance and the resulting acute energy shortage have brought waves of fear crashing down on the words and ideas people use to comfort themselves when they are faced with unwelcome, unavoidable change, doubt, complexity and mystery. Stories that once were told to provide hope, strength and patience now spark dread and helplessness in the storyteller. In short, our stories have little in common with Odysseus', which gave him the strength to find his way home–through twenty years of twists and turns, through bravery, trickery and bloodshed.

Another important point about these stories: They are irrelevant. Change quickly washes away context. For example, a valid observation about your health or mental outlook that was made six months ago, let alone six years ago, has lost all but the slightest shadow of its original meaning. Change is so pervasive–from the external stimulus of a changing environment to the inner landscape that results from the body's response. Stories are generally woven together using incidents, episodes and crises to form an overview. The product is then used to explain the past. In the hands of someone with a negative mindset it becomes an encyclopedia of excuses, an autobiography of failure. Worse, it is held up as an indispensable way to prepare for the future and manage outcomes that will make us or break us. Stories such as these are in the same league as the utterances of false prophets.

A ten-year-old story is worthless. The client who brings it to us is not the same person. He may try to be, thereby creating havoc through poor choices, frustration and anger that he represents.

For roughly my first twenty years as a postural therapist, I considered the stories my clients brought with them on their initial visits to the clinic to be, at best, a package of clues that explained why they were in pain or, at worst, a social nicety that allowed us to build a solid working relationship. I hardly noticed the obvious: The clients who made the most progress on correcting their musculoskeletal dysfunctions were the ones who readily put their stories aside. They focused on how they were feeling at that moment, not on the memory of how it felt when they were told at age fourteen that they had scoliosis or other chronic conditions. As I encouraged them to change their posture and range of motion, they felt the pain diminish and function return. The old story ceased to matter as a new autobiography took shape.

I concluded that the best way to go was to get the storytelling over the sooner the better, and to encourage the client to pay attention to how they feel—not to how they felt. And that worked, except for a small percentage that used their stories to explain why they couldn't possibly get well. Frustrated, I would often—way too often—shoot holes in their story to force them to give it up (and prove how smart I was).

After much soul-searching, I decided that the only solution was to devise a way for the client to change his or her story without being forced to admit that they were changing it. Reworking the heath care paradigm one story at a time was extremely daunting until I realized that all the problematic stories were fear-based; furthermore, each fit into one of only three broad variations that can be deconstructed like this:

- *I've been to everyone and tried everything. Nothing works. I don't know where to turn. Help me if you can, but you probably can't. This is not my fault.*
- *I'm determined to figure this out, and to take control. What's your solution? There are so many moving parts. Your recommendations are in conflict with other schools of thought. Have you considered...? I need another opinion. Are you aware of this new study?*

- *What makes you so smart? None of this stuff works. It's all a scam. Nobody has an answer. Prove it. I don't feel any different.*

I hope that captures the emotional and behavioral predilections of the three without holding them up to ridicule or suggesting that one or another is more or less desirable. I do not want to offend you—because you may fit one of these categories. If so, your fears, triggered by musculoskeletal system imbalance and the consequent critical energy shortage, are expressed by one of the three storytelling variations.

All three are afraid to go inward to obtain and marshal the resources needed to recover or sustain the storyteller's health. The stories were self-created to shield them from fear and to allow them to go on living in the presence of it. The storytellers inadvertently wall themselves off by denying personal responsibility, insatiably seeking new facts and treatment options without making commitments, or unintentionally coating themselves in the Teflon of cynicism to stand aloof on the sidelines.

Your own story is much richer, deeper and meatier than my abbreviated outline, but if you can feel your way to the essence of the story I believe you will find a platform from which, together, you and I can work to restore your postural balance, your limitless energy, and your perfect health.

In the next three chapters I will describe the musculoskeletal markers of the three storylines and personality types. There are physical and functional characteristics for each. You'll be able to pick them out of a crowd; better yet, you'll be able to look in the mirror and recognize yourself. Then I will present menus of E-cises (Egoscue-cises) that can help recover musculoskeletal system balance, tailored to work with your specific story and type.

Rather than falling back on your story to explain why you can't restore your balance—*too busy, too late, runs in the family, birth defect, Egoscue's too pushy*—you can really do this.

Really.

You are enough.

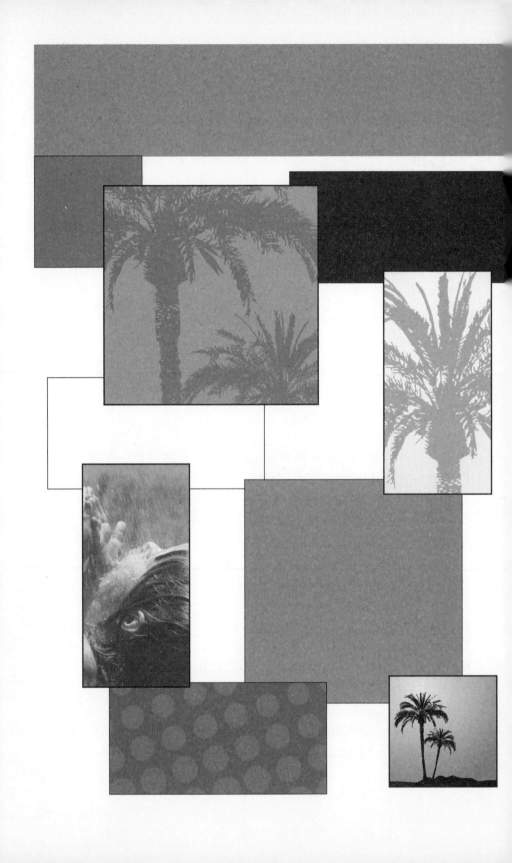

Blame Blam

Never explain, never complain is a pretty good rule, yet I'm going to break half of it. I'm not a complainer, but when I blow it the least I can do is give you a heads-up about what didn't go as well as it should have.

In my first book, *The Egoscue Method of Health through Motion*, I described the outward physical characteristics of three categories of musculoskeletal system dysfunction, and offered guidance on how readers could easily figure out whether they fit into Conditions I, II or III. The idea was to provide a process for self-diagnosis that would set the stage for the next step, do-it-yourself postural therapy that addressed the specifics of each condition. As I wrote at the time—if you know what to look for, musculoskeletal misalignment and imbalance are easy to spot.

Strike Three

What surprised me, however, was that many people couldn't do it. In particular, my description of what to look for and the accompanying drawings of typical Condition III's caused so much consternation only the most intrepid readers could bring themselves to gaze into the mirror and admit they looked that bad! Condition II's were slightly better at self-diagnosis but not by much.

Both II's and III's, even if they were in horrible pain, tended to chose Condition I, which led them to follow an E-cise menu that didn't work as well.

Amazingly, I still get rave reviews for the book. People call the Del Mar clinic out of the blue to tell me how good those E-cises make them feel. When I ask a few questions about what's currently going on with their body and hear answers that indicate that they are classic, industrial-strength Condition III's, I've learned to say, "Go to the E-cises for Condition III—don't look at the pictures or read the description, just try the E-cise menu." Often they sound shocked that I would even think of linking them by inference to Condition III. I fear that some of them put down the phone and, convinced they misunderstood, go straight back to Condition I. There's no harm done (on the contrary, a lot of help is delivered nevertheless), other than they are not getting the full benefit of the Method.

The sad truth is that today, more than ever, my unvarnished description of Condition III in *The Egoscue Method* is what most Americans and most affluent and middle-class people around the world look like and hurt like. Tragically, that look of imbalance and musculoskeletal misalignment has become the new normal. When the old normal walks by, a rarer and rarer occurrence, he or she seems strange.

Sorry. What I intended as a brief preamble to the remaining chapters has turned out to be longer and more involved than I'd like it to be. No postural therapy program can be designed to fit all comers and conditions. But there are three broad categories—yup, still three—of readily observable musculoskeletal system conditions that are accompanied by overt behavioral patterns that are expressed as actions, attitudes, and emotions. I call them 'AAE patterns'.

To put it more plainly, it is not the postures that matter—it's your head. To help you make a self-diagnosis, I don't have to show you any examples of dysfunction. And to that I say Hallelujah! There's no need to scare you with lurid depictions of desperate people who are about to crash and burn. Instead I will help you feel what's going on in your head, in your heart and in your body's core systems that monitor and operate this amazing thing that we so casually refer to as human health. Best of all, you won't have to take my word for it. You know more about your body than any expert because you feel it and they don't.

I started this book by asking—"How do you feel?" However, some people—perhaps I'm talking about you—can't answer that question because one of the three most common AAE patterns is disrupting their ability to get an accurate reading from their emotional feedback loop.

Example: J.B.'s back was hurting when he came to see me a couple of years ago at the San Diego clinic. He told me right off, "I've got a herniated disk."

> **Easy Rider**
>
> The individual vertebrae of the spine ride on cushions—spongy disks that resemble jelly donuts—that act as shock absorbers. Imbalance and misalignment result in the weight of the upper torso and head squeezing down on the disks unevenly to cause the "jelly" to either bulge from between the vertebrae or rupture (it actually pops like a balloon and the filling oozes out). Either way, the result is a painful nerve impingement.

Okay. It is not a nice thing to have. I asked him to stand pigeon-toed with both cheeks of the buttocks, and the lower and upper backs against the wall. Try it yourself: Level the chin and make sure the back of your heads is against the wall, otherwise there is a tendency for the head and neck to come forward and down. Now put the shoulders against the wall.

"How's it feel now?"

"Still hurts."

"Really?"

"Yeah, really. I can show you the X-ray of the disk."

"But it still hurts? No change?"

"Of course."

I didn't argue with J.B., but I knew that the pigeon-toed stance temporarily repositioned his hips and in so doing moved the affected vertebrae off the distended disk to free the jammed nerve. Without the impingement, the magnitude of the pain had to decrease. While there might have been an echo of tenderness, the worst of the pain went away almost immediately. The reaction didn't surprise me, though. J.B.'s feelings were being distorted by his default AAE pattern. He was a big, strong, courageous guy, yet fear had switched off his ability to accurately assess what was going on in his back.

Pain is not a disease, not an injury, not even an effect of aging. Pain is a symptom; in J.B.'s case, a symptom of postural imbalance. Not the only one; there were many others that produced little or no pain at all. The way he sliced a golf ball, for instance (pain-free as long as you weren't in the line

---

Making Choices

Since J.B.'s visit I have changed my approach. Instead of starting with a demonstration of how postural balance can switch off the pain symptom, we have a discussion of whether the client wants a cure or treatment. Surprisingly, about 1 in 20 opt for treatment (i.e., mostly pain suppression).

of fire) and the contortions he went through to get in and out of his car.[12] Symptoms are irrelevant—go for a cure. Cures come about only when the bullet of intervention is aimed at, and hits, the actual cause of a condition. Shooting innocent bystanders usually serves only to create collateral damage and costly medical bills.

> ### Got Your Back
> Favorite symptomatic treatments of herniated disks are removing the disk in conjunction with fusing the adjoining vertebrae, or trimming away the ruptured disk material. No matter what, the spine is still unbalanced and unevenly squeezing the remaining disks. Fusing the vertebrae worsens the imbalance and creates stress on the shoulders, hips, knees and ankles; and snipping off the protruding disk material probably means you'll be having a lot of recurring back surgery.

For J.B. the cause was lack of energy. His back pain and postural imbalances were symptoms of an energy crisis that always occurs when the body is left unplugged. Just as the ice cream stored in your kitchen freezer will melt if the electricity goes out for a couple of hours, when the body goes off-line and loses contact with the universal power grid, it too melts. Musculoskeletal form and function are quickly lost without a constant flow of high wavelength energy. Why? Death dematerializes living tissue. Only the energy endures forever. Short of death, the early, obvious and progressive stages of dematerialization are the body's means of warning us that something is happening that in many cases (far more than we think) is within our power to substantially affect. By ignoring the message or merely addressing pain symptoms with pain

---

[12] J.B. used to drive a low-slung Italian job but the struggle of lowering himself into the driver's seat caused serious pain. Eventually he sold it and bought something more sedate. But even his new luxury sedan was a challenge to J.B. until he got his functional posture back.

killers, joint replacement and other forms of surgery (treatment), the most important message of all is lost—*Lack of energy
is killing you, and it is time for you to change the stimulus.*

This is one of the most important points in the book. Your
musculoskeletal system is the trip-wire that sets off the first of
many alarms. When our earliest ancestors first showed up on
dry land they didn't have the technological tools to rat around
inside the body, surf the bloodstream, test drive the immune
system, and the like. Instead, they relied on simply being aware
of seemingly superficial changes that took place on the body's
surface or close to it: *My left foot is turned out instead of
pointing straight ahead; my spear-chucking arm seems stiff;* or
*I'm having trouble keeping pace with my favorite hunting
companions.* Those folks weren't rocket scientists, yet they
were smart enough to recognize that something had changed.
Nothing comes of nothing. They learned to either alter the
stimulus that was causing the change (finding a dry place to
sleep in monsoon season is the 10,000-year-old man's way of
altering stimulus), or they lived with the consequences, which
often meant dying sooner rather than later. Natural selection
favored those who took action based on awareness, and their
biological heirs are still blessed with the trip-wire provided by
the musculoskeletal system.

J.B. has come a long way, but he has misplaced his awareness. If I could have waved a magic wand to instantly restore
J.B.'s postural balance, his energy levels would have quickly
topped off. What prevented that—aside from my wand being in
the repair shop to have its abracadabra generator rebuilt—was
that he was afraid to accept the idea that something as simple
as postural balance was the answer. He resisted treatment in
order to keep pursuing what he regarded as more plausible
and more reassuring facts.

In reality, J.B. found more comfort in seeking and collecting new facts, theories, information and such than he got

from living truly pain-free. Fact-collecting is a common AAE pattern (remember–*actions, attitudes, emotions*). J.B.'s body was aware of the dangerous shortage of energy and informed him of the situation with a variety of messages, including pain symptoms and such non-pain symptoms as fatigue, irritability and lack of focus. But his thinking mind had outsmarted his feeling mind by persuading him that he could exert control over these symptoms by using his high IQ and practical experience. Like most fact collectors, however, the search for another set of new facts precludes fact-based actions. What's the point? The new new facts will blow away the old new facts.

Ready, set, go! He chased facts when in reality all he had to do was stand there and feel the energy being renewed and health restored as his body was temporarily brought back into balance. I'll return to J.B. in a moment; meantime, I want to stop here briefly to deal more directly with the invisible elephant in the room: physical limitation, the Big Foot of postural therapy. I've already discussed the importance of an individual's story. The story frames what would otherwise be a meaningless jumble of events, incidents and sensations. The various pieces of a narrative give meaning and value to the life it represents. A story may be true or false, and in a general sense is neither good nor bad. It just is. Yet a story infused by forebodings of physical limitation and what they portend has the power to interfere with your feeling mind. As a creature of the night it is disturbing.

Here's how: J.B. sees the world as a dangerously complicated place. Consequently, he must discover what makes it tick. He searches diligently for facts that will give him the ability to manage the present, predict and prepare for the future, and survive. It is a never-ending quest because new facts are constantly trumping old facts. As a result, he never needs to make a choice and run the risk of being wrong, which in a complicated, dangerous world could be lethal. Hence, J.B.'s story is crippled by his compulsion to keep collecting facts.

The second of these AAE patterns is skepticism. Like fact-collecting, it is also driven by anxiety about physical limitation, which lodges in the emotional catacombs when the musculoskeletal system first experiences a gap in its repertoire of movement. L.J., a child psychologist, freely admitted she was a complete skeptic about anyone and anything who claimed to solve problems or accomplish objectives. She was always on guard against being conned. For her, everyone was suspected of having a fishy, hidden agenda. It was L.J.'s job to find it. Acute skepticism protected her from ever making an affirmative decision, and hence she was never responsible for her own health.

The third AAE pattern is pessimism, the most extreme form of fear of physical limitation. T.N. worked in pessimism the way some artists work in watercolors. He sought help from dozens of health care practitioners, was always willing to try another therapeutic program but believed that they would fail because he didn't deserve to succeed.

I am about to introduce three chapters that will offer more information on these patterns, including recommendations for postural therapy programs that have demonstrated the ability to overcome them. The catch is I don't know which one of them is affecting you. It's going to have to be your call, your decision.

I can't knock experts who are ready, willing and unable to assume responsibility for your health and then pretend that I am an exception to the rule. The road from here on belongs to you. I've struggled to keep the three patterns from appearing to be other forms of the infamous Condition III, so daunting that you and other readers would shy away from making a choice and taking action to restore your musculoskeletal system to balance, and thereby miss the chance to plug back into the universal energy grid before it is too late.

Notice that I've avoided linking the patterns closely to an individual. It doesn't matter who you are, what you do, if you are young, old, male or female. I used initials rather than names and offered a very sketchy personal profile in the examples to avoid the pitfall of implying that I'm talking only about certain people, say professional women, jocks or Type A's. I hope that you won't identify with the example or, on the other hand, decide that I'm talking about someone else.

Read all three of the chapters and, by the feel of it, not the think of it, decide which of them may be affecting your ability to live pain-free. Try the postural therapy program for that specific fear pattern. Again, by the feel of it, not the think of it, decide if the program works. If not, reread the chapters (or the entire book) and try another program. You may need to try all three. Take your time; stay in the moment.

Just ask yourself—How do I feel?

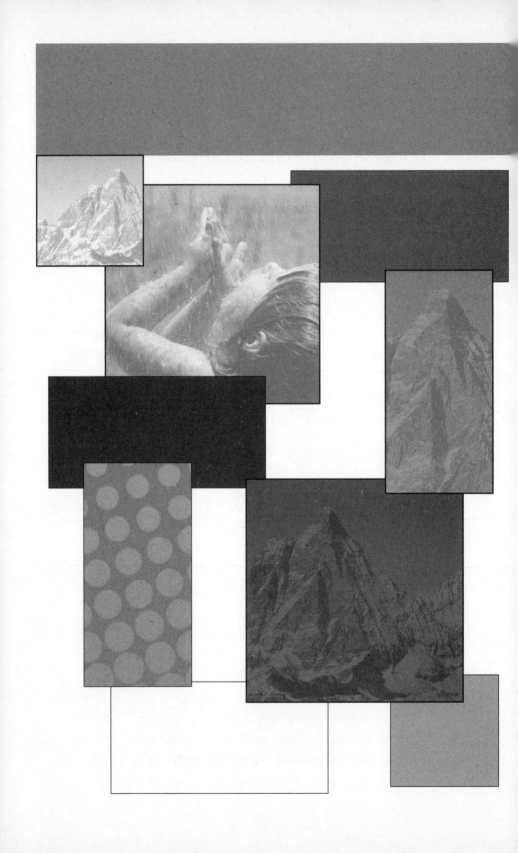

The Weight of Evidence

In the last chapter I promised to introduce you to three personality types that are the most threatened by musculoskeletal system imbalance. The place to start is with the fact collectors. Of the three personality types, fact collectors are my favorite. It's not that I dislike the others. It comes down to a simple matter of recognizing that what they require–a steady supply of new facts–is quite easy to deliver as long as those of us who are trying to achieve pain-free lives are careful to distinguish between external facts and internal facts.

The human musculoskeletal system is a symphony of facts, but as obsessed as they are with collecting them, fact collectors like J.B. (who was featured in the preceding chapter, so if you skipped over it you might want to backtrack a little) are conditioned to gather only facts from external sources that legitimize, sanction and officially confirm that what the collector sees, smells, tastes, touches and hears is the real deal. As a result, J.B. rarely looked within himself to discover and authenticate facts. This is, to say the least, a problem.

By establishing a higher authority to validate facts, J.B. disenfranchised himself. Humans have a gift for discerning the real from the unreal, truth from falsehood, the genuine from the fake. If we didn't, our species would have become extinct thousands of years ago. There's far too much quicksand, thin ice and slipperiness in the dark and dangerous places of our native habitat for creatures devoid of acutely sensitive preternatural survival skills to flourish the way we have without a reasonably effective means for screening out the phony and the fallacious.

Thanks to your ancestors, who learned the hard way to live on and rule over this planet, you are nobody's fool. Before there was a thinking mind, there was—and still is—an aware mind that allows humans to quickly distinguish things that are promising from those that are perilous by accessing subjective, road-tested standards imbedded deep in our sensory apparatus. Objective facts have little or no relevance to the aware mind, which is tuned to a different frequency. It doesn't give a damn about the think of things. Subjective facts rule. Gathered over the course of time like scar tissue, they are a potent distillation drawn from the raw ingredients of personal experiences. What drips out of the spigot is 1,000-proof feeling.

Fact collectors have lost contact with the aware mind. To them, a fact must have a pedigree, a seal of approval; otherwise, it is an opinion of limited value. J.B. and his cohorts come to the Egoscue clinics with MRIs, X-rays, file folders stuffed full of medical records and vocabularies bristling with

Latinate jargon. I used to refuse to look at the material, preferring instead to directly observe the individual's posture. But I was inadvertently denying full fact-hood to the client's condition by treating the official documentation like ... like opinions. Just as a connoisseur of pre-Columbian pottery would be put off if I refused to admire their treasures, the fact collectors were affronted by my indifference toward their precious authenticated facts. Now, after a good twenty or more years of being obtuse, I make a point of reviewing the records and agreeing that, *Yes, the X-ray shows the disk is ruptured* or *No doubt about it, that knee is badly swollen.*

Story attempts to provide meaning. By shaping a narrative out of all the bits and pieces of existence—here's the beginning, the middle, and the end—storytellers try to create coherence out of confusion. J.B.'s story, the one that helps him make sense of his life and calms his fears, is built around a core belief that he can be safe (or safer) as long as he can put a wall of facts between himself and the predator that is stalking him; e.g., not grizzlies and tigers, but limitation, illness, pain, aging, death. A fact collector believes that if he can assemble all the "true" facts about his situation, a solution will emerge. In other words, the story is a classic *whodunit* with the fact collector cast as the heroic private eye.

Facts become all-important. People like J.B. shop for facts, savor facts, trade in dented and scratched old facts for bright, shiny new facts. It doesn't take long for fact-finding to become a substitute for action. Instead of making a decision and following through on it to change the conditions that are causing or contributing to the pain or another symptom, fact collectors seek different sets of facts that are obligingly generated by medical science, the pharmaceutical industry, and experts of every sort. They are free to choose a fact to their liking and use it as a basis for treatment or cure—and that's fine. However, most often it is an excuse to avoid treatment or cure altogether, since a new fact is waiting just around the next corner. Another tendency is to passively submit to someone else's opinion on what is best because they are offering a convincing presentation of the facts coincidental to a symptom becoming too painful or unpleasant to be endured.

My challenge as a postural therapist is to figure out a way to get the inner voice of the aware mind within earshot of their inner facts. Once that happens, the need for another set of new, externally generated facts usually fades away. Feelings are better than facts. A balanced musculoskeletal system feels right (and it is!). By offering J.B. a few E-cises to stabilize his posture, I could then ask, "How does that feel?" and get a useful answer.

"It feels a little better."

"Good. You still have a ruptured disk—that's a fact."

"That's true."

"But these E-cises affected the pain—that also seems to be a fact, doesn't it?"

"Yeah."

"Does it make sense to you to continue the E-cises and see what happens?"

"Well, the E-cises do seem to work. The low back feels different."

Most fact collectors will go home from the clinic, think about their first visit and come back with a couple of other facts. Maybe they've called their doctor or gone on the Internet. The Web is teeming with facts. I've learned not to argue with those external facts. The best approach is to return to the inner facts. "How do you feel?"

"A little better. But my left knee has started to hurt again."

"What's that tell you?"

"Maybe I'm standing up straighter, and the knee isn't used to that."

"If you are, we are impacting the dysfunction, jump-starting disused muscles. Let's see if we can build on this progress. Want to give it a shot?"

The Role of Energy Depletion

I am not asking him to believe my facts. I don't have the slightest interest in being in the external fact business. I'm inviting him to believe his inner facts and to link them to the gradually receding pain and other symptoms like the knee. I used to think that postural balance—even partially restored balance—felt so good that clients would always immediately respond. But I now believe that when high wavelength energy is depleted it may take several tries to get it back to a level that is sufficient to completely switch off the craving for external facts. Awareness requires energy. When you can't go there, it usually means that musculoskeletal system imbalance has drained your energy supply to the extent that it is almost empty. Yet by just making a brief reconnect in the form of a simple balancing E-cise, energy starts flowing again. A lot of energy.

Even so, a fact collector will be tempted to stop and carefully scrutinize her vast fact collection, comparing the newcomers to the old favorites. This can be frustrating. Instead of moving forward, she digs in her heels, seeks to question everything, and arranges and rearranges the facts in order to assign more value to some and lesser importance to others. Hairs are split and angels dance on the heads of pins. It helps to have an abundance of patience; otherwise, fact collectors start to seem unreasonably rigid and prone to willfully obstructing a cure.

Indeed, rigidity is the overarching postural and emotional characteristic of fact collectors. They are tight, stiff, tense, constricted. The facts don't give them any wiggle room. Life isn't much fun. When they look to the right or left they cannot just move their head; the whole body rotates. If you removed the driver-side mirror from his car before his cure, J.B. would have been unable to glance over his shoulder at the traffic approaching from the left rear. His peripheral vision was poor; when walking he plodded along. There was little spontaneity or variation in stride or tempo.

When he first came to the clinic and stood sideways next to a ceiling-to-floor plumb-line, J.B.'s ankle was on the line but the knee, hip, upper torso, shoulder, neck and ear fell in front of the line. He thought he was standing straight but was actually raked forward like the bow of a ship. The body's internal sensors read the posture and concluded that he was only a few degrees away from toppling forward. Red alert! Muscles were contracted from head to foot and joints locked to hold the body upright, sacrificing lateral movement and rotational flexibility in the interest of keeping him from going horizontal.

Bear in mind this is not routine posture; it is the posture of crisis and calamity. Whenever a fact collector is on his feet, the internal alarm bells are ringing big-time, the nervous system is fired up, and energy is being poured into vital physiological processes that for all they know are about to be asked to function in a state of emergency. And our guy is only walking from his easy chair to the bathroom! Ironically, most fact collectors aren't couch potatoes. They keep fairly active. I see them rigid and running, rigid and inline skating, rigid and golfing, and rigidly playing a variety of weekend sports—because the facts say they need to keep fit. They also frequently hurt themselves, at which point they start collecting facts to prove that running when you're over forty is hard on the knees, that tennis rackets stress your elbow, and golf is hard on the back.

However, those are external facts. Restoring balance by just ten or fifteen percent delivers an instant energy payoff. By accumulating high wavelength energy rather than running a deficit, even the most dedicated fact collector quickly starts to feel better. Once postural balance is restored, he loses the urgent compulsion to grab at external facts to explain his sense of panic and foreboding. His aware mind is reinvigorated. J.B. and others like him can live in the moment, drawing pleasure and peace of mind where he once hustled after facts to compensate for not being present.

Are you a fact collector? Before you answer, mull over the following questions:

- How do you make decisions? Fast or slow? Is it easy or do you agonize?
- Are you prone to second-guessing your decisions?
- Do you frequently change your mind?
- How do you rate yourself as a decision-maker?
- Are you afraid of making mistakes?
- What was your best decision?
- What was your worst decision?
- Are you stubborn?
- Are you a perfectionist?
- Who is the smartest person you know?
- Do you welcome responsibility?
- Are you rigid?
- Do you go by the book?
- Are there decisions you prefer to avoid?

So? Or do you need more facts?
Here's one–balance. Try it. Please.

E-cise Menu for Fact Collectors

Static Back

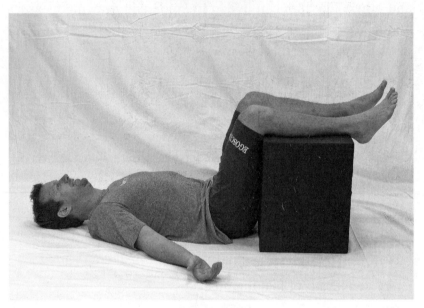

Figure 10-E1

This E-cise uses the force of gravity to settle the hips, back and shoulders to the floor and put them into a neutral position. Lie on your back with both legs bent at right angles and resting on a chair, a bench or a block. Rest your hands on your stomach or the floor, below shoulder level, with palms up. Let the back settle into the floor. Breathe from your diaphragm. That is, do stomach breathing—the abdominal muscles should rise as you inhale and fall as you exhale. Stay in this position for ten minutes. Relax.

Knee-pillow Squeezes in Static Back

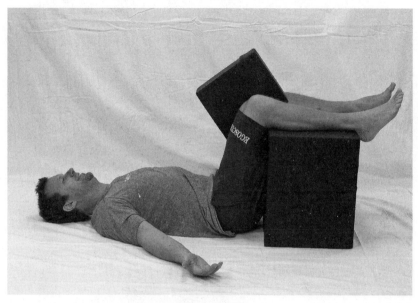

Figure 10-E2

Stay in the static back. Widen your feet to allow a fat pillow or a foam block to fit between your knees. Squeeze the knees together using the inside (abductor) muscles of the thighs. Give the pillow a firm squeeze, then release. Don't tighten your abdominal muscles. Do three sets of twenty.

Hip Lifts

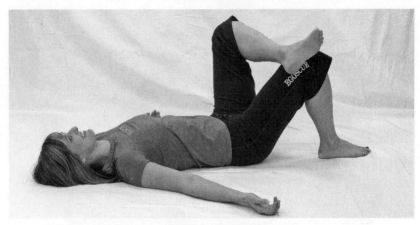

Figure 10-E5 (a)

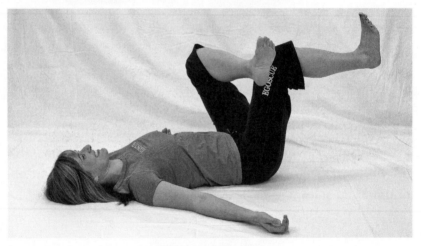

Figure 10-E6 (b)

This E-cise repositions and levels your hips. Lie on your back with both knees bent and your feet flat on the floor. Cross your left ankle on your right knee, and press your left knee away from your body. While maintaining this position, lift your right foot off the floor, bringing both legs toward your chest. Make sure your hips stay squared and on the floor, that your left knee is still pressing out, that your right leg is in line with your right shoulder and that your hips are still on the floor. After one minute switch the legs and repeat on the other side.

Hip Crossover

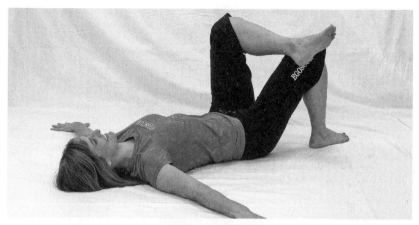

Figure 10-E7 (a)

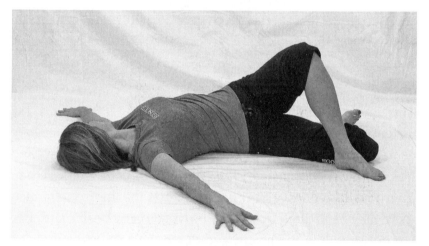

Figure 10-E8 (b)

This E-cise counteracts hip rotation on both sides. Lie on your back with your knees bent and your feet flat on the floor. Place your arms on the floor at shoulder level. Cross your left ankle over your right knee, and rotate the ankle/knee combination to the floor to your right. Turn your head so that you are look-ing to the left, and relax your shoulders. Press your left knee away from your body with the left hip musculature. Switch the ankle/knee crossover, and repeat on the opposite side.

Frog

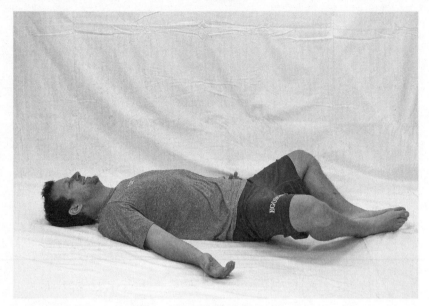

Figure 10-E3

This E-cise positions the pelvis symmetrically left to right. Lie on your back with your knees bent. Make sure your feet are centered in the middle of your body, and let your knees and legs fall away to the sides. Put the soles of your feet together. Your low back does not need to be flat on the floor, and in fact, there may be an arch due to the hips' changing position. Relax. Do not press the thighs out and down. Feel the stretch in the inner thighs and groin. Three minutes.

Standing Arm Circles

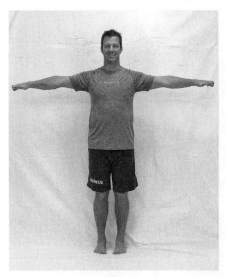   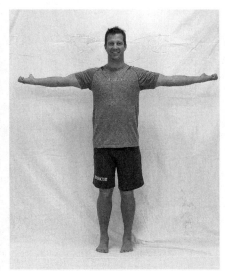

Figure 10-E20 (a)   **Figure 10-E21 (b)**

This E-cise strengthens the muscles of the upper back that are involved with the shoulders' ball-and-socket function. Stand facing a mirror with your feet parallel, about hips-width apart, your arms at your sides. Curl your fingertips into the pads of each palm (the fleshy area at the base of the fingers), and point your thumbs straight out. This hand position, called the "golfer's grip," is imperative to the success of this E-cise. Squeeze your shoulder blades together, and bring your arms out to the sides at shoulder level, elbows straight. With your palms facing down, thumbs pointed forward, circle up and forward for thirty repetitions. With your arms still out at shoulder level, palms up, circle up and back for thirty repetitions. Remember to keep your wrists, arms, and elbows straight with the shoulder blades squeezed together. Don't contract your stomach muscles—the circles must come from the shoulders. Keep your neck and head back. Do thirty forward and thirty back.

Standing Quad Stretch

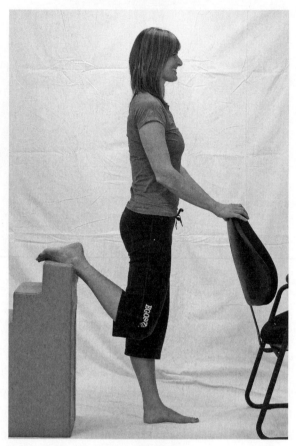

Figure 10-E28

Hip rotation shuts the quads off; this E-cise turns them back on. Stand on one foot and bend the other leg back, placing the top of the foot on a block or chair seat (the elevation should be somewhere between the bottom of the buttock and your hipline). The amount of stretch depends on how high your foot is propped. Keep your hips and shoulders square and your knees even, and tuck your hips under to feel the stretch. Hold on to something for balance. One side will probably be tighter than the other but do not vary the foot elevation from side to side. One minute a side; use the same elevation for both.

Cats & Dogs

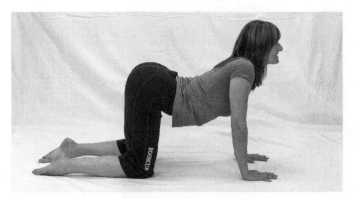

Figure 10-E11 (a)

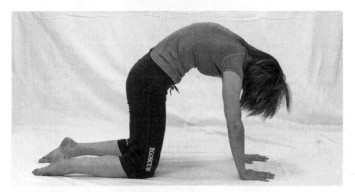

Figure 10-E12 (b)

This E-cise works the hips, spine, shoulders and neck in coordinated flexion-extension. Get down on the floor on your hands and knees. Make sure your knees are aligned with your hips, your wrists and your shoulders; your lower legs should be parallel with each other and with your hips. Make sure your weight is distributed evenly. Smoothly round your back as your head curls under to create a curve that runs from the buttocks to the neck—this is the cat with an arched back. Smoothly sway the back down while bringing the head up—now the perky dog. Make these two moves flow continuously back and forth rather than allowing them to be distinct and choppy. Ten repetitions; one cat and one dog count as one.

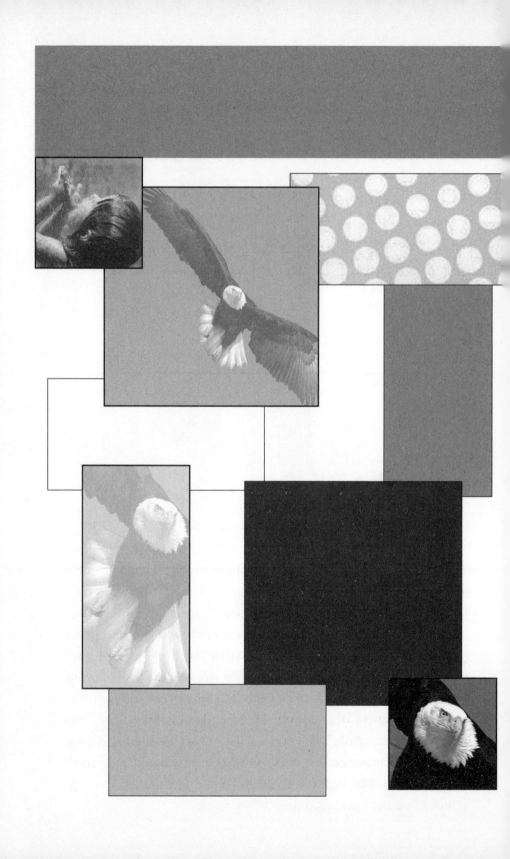

The Skeptic and the Gospel of Doubt

Read any good autobiographies lately?

You have if you so much as looked into the mirror today or glanced at a passing stranger. Posture is autobiography, an external embodiment of our inner state. It records and explains what we did, and why it was done to become who we are.

Your distinctive postural profile exposes all secrets of commission, omission and submission. Don't worry—the evidence is not admissible in a court of law. Yet it is extraordinarily useful if you want to know why you've been unable to be truly pain-free, depression-free, self-doubt-free; why resolutions to diet, get in shape, gain control over self-destructive habits and the like have come to naught.

The second personality type that I am going to discuss is the skeptic, who is fated to live a life of total contradiction: He or she believes only in doubt.

The skeptic expects to be cheated. The world, he is sure, is full of bandits, incompetents and hidden pitfalls. Only the vigilant, the canny, the tough survive. He armor-plates his ego and refuses to be lured out into the open where his superior IQ might be defeated by trickery and bad luck.

Skeptics are indeed smart. Quick-witted and well educated, they can be fun to be around. But there is more darkness than light in their story. Their cynical expectations rob them of their primary power and their greatest gifts—positive energy, joy and peace of mind. When they come to the clinic, the typical skeptic is in pain. There is a postural condition (most likely) that has left them unbalanced and energy-depleted. Without being directly conscious of it, they are afraid—afraid of illness, injury, aging, limitation. Their story is intended to make the fear easier to bear, yet it actually makes things worse. Much worse.

Their story is a form of absolution—self-forgiveness and self-soothing: *I am not to blame; I was cheated by the system; I had no choice; I inherited my grandfather's high blood pressure.* There are many variations. Fair enough, but the story goes a bit farther, and thereby topples off the edge: *Since I am clearly not to blame, maybe I won't be punished.* Our egos lash us when we fall short of perfection. A perfect person does not get sick or injured. Of course that's nonsense, but our inner scold, critic and all-around harpy bedevils us with a steady stream of backseat driving.

For a skeptic it is a heavy burden. She substitutes a doubting, blame-shifting attitude for awareness and acceptance of personal responsibility. It seems safer and easier to hide out behind tough, know-it-all negativity than to face up to the task of recovering lost balance, retrieving lost knowing and rediscovering a never truly lost yet often never awakened, fully energized peace of mind. However daunting it may appear—you can do it, you are enough—we, you, me, all of us were made from the ground up to accomplish this task.

As a postural therapist, skeptics used to give me fits. They have always been among the brightest of my clients, yet when they had completed an item from their menu of balancing E-cises and I asked how they felt, often the answer was, "Feels the same." I could see with one quick glance that the E-cises had done their work—the shoulder, hip, whatever it was that had been misaligned was at least beginning to move back into its proper place. It surprised and baffled me that they didn't feel it. For many years, I assumed they were either willfully, perversely refusing to cooperate or that some physiological mechanism was overriding what they should have been feeling.

By being patient and forcing myself to listen and to observe closely, I detected that skeptics indeed felt the change; even so, they did not trust it enough to acknowledge to me or to themselves that they were aware of the feeling. What they felt came and went too fast, or didn't stand out against the background noise and distractions. It seemed like a fleeting, half-remembered, half-forgotten dream. I had to find a way to make those quick flashes cohere into an enduring awareness.

A client, L.J., gave me the first breakthrough. There was pain in his right hip. I asked him to stand on his right foot with the left leg bent at the knee so that the left foot could be stretched back to allow the toes to hook behind him on the front edge of a waist-high countertop.[13] He had been standing that way for three minutes. When I asked him to put both feet back on the floor and move his right hip a little to see if it still hurt, he muttered flippantly, "Dream on." As soon as his foot was off the countertop, though, his eyes widened in disbelief.

"Well?"

"Same."

It was a complete lie. Actually, it was an incomplete lie—the eyes revealed the truth. The E-cise had repositioned his hip, putting the pelvis in a level (right to left) position instead dropping away to the right, which left the hip joint grinding in the socket. Rather than challenge him, I surrendered, or seemed to. "I guess you've stumped me." I went on to say something to the effect that what the clinic was offering just wasn't right for him and that we would refund his money. L.J. immediately rejected the offer and suggested that I was being too hasty and that maybe, now that he had a chance to think about it, he could feel a change in his hip.

That was the buy-in I was looking for. Instead of closing the sale, I borrowed a little of his cynicism: "Just got lucky, I guess." And that response endures to this day whenever we deal with a skeptic in one of our clinics. I advise my therapists not to attack the story—ride it home in triumph. *Just got lucky....* is okay with me, since I know the lucky part is having the human musculoskeletal system. Very soon the skeptic—make that the former skeptic—will too.

---

[13] If you try this E-cise and have trouble getting the back leg into position, use the seat of a chair instead of a countertop. Stand straight with your head and shoulders back. Keep the hips even side-to-side (not rotated) and level. Use the back of another chair to help keep your balance. If you are having problems with this one it confirms that you need a lot of work on your hips.

I have always suspected that even self-proclaimed cynics (skeptics on steroids) never completely succeed in fooling themselves into believing their own cynicism. They are actually seeking confirmation in the form of road-tested personal experience that it is safe to have faith. Instinctively, all of us know that having faith in one's self is the source of peace of mind. Knowing that we are enough is indeed enough. By agreeing to play along with their cynicism as it pertains to every human being's role in co-creating their health, and by not immediately requiring them to buy into a need for an unshakable faith in self, I am briefly sharing their story, their secret, but also giving them a chance to experience musculoskeletal system balance and renewed energy. In time (and it won't be long!), being present and aware of what's taking place causes the cynical story to fall away to reveal the truth.

Skeptics look like they are moving sideways—and they are. They use their wits and deep distrust to slip around obstacles. A shoulder or a hip, often both, are rotated forward and to the left which gives skeptics, both male and female, an appearance of drifting off at an angle as they walk forward. And they would drift without some artful counter-torquing by their knees, by the sockets of the hip joints, and by head fakes (tilting, turning and thrusting) that serve as rudders to keep them on course.

Am I saying that there is a skeptic musculoskeletal system type that is paired with the personality type?

Exactly. (The same is also true for the other two personality types.)

Our posture reveals how we move. How we move is who we are. Skeptics try to protect their heart; both as a working pump and a locus of the spirit. Yes, spirit. I am not at all reluctant to think of the heart as being the place where love, courage and generosity dwell. And I'll bet that if I asked you and my other readers to draw a heart, many would, without giving a second thought, sketch the cutesy Hallmark version.

Only an anatomy geek prefers a Valentine's Day card shaped like a cross between an eggplant and an old four-barrel carburetor.

Expressions like "pure hearts," "strong stomach," and "sweet tooth," are rooted in awareness that the body and its various parts are full participants in our spiritual life.

A skeptic feels extremely vulnerable advancing straight at the world with his precious heart exposed; consequently, he adopts a defensive posture by rotating the pelvis and the upper torso so that the heart is being shielded by the shoulders and ribcage. This rotation is the crux of musculoskeletal system dysfunction. It disrupts the vertical load-bearing alignment that allows us to move forward smoothly in a straight line, change direction without losing our balance, hop on one foot, carry a load and, in general, to easily get around without mishap and injury. The alignment and interaction of four horizontal parallel planes created by the shoulders, the hips, the knees and the ankles/feet combined with two vertical parallel planes formed by the paired load joints (i.e., right shoulder, right hip, right knee and right ankle/foot, and left shoulder, left hip, left knee and left ankle/foot) constitute a precisely calibrated, invisible scaffolding that makes us one of the most mobile creatures on earth.

Take a Plane

If the musculoskeletal system is fully functional, your major load-bearing joints are in horizontal and vertical planar alignment. A plane is a boundless flat surface of infinite extent and no thickness, encompassing three or more points not on a straight line.

By rotating her shoulders and hips, a skeptic disrupts balance. To avoid falling, she resorts to a variety of dodges that strain muscles, damage joints and severely limit her range of movement. At the same time, it creates a distinct, misaligned, non-vertical posture that is mistakenly regarded as an individual physical expression of family traits, lifestyle, random selection or aging.

When you lose your vertical and horizontal integrity, the posture displayed is a symptom of illness. It may not hurt yet, but it soon will. The dysfunctional posture is interfering with the body's need for healthy, unrestricted movement and it is relentlessly undermining vital physiological processes.

Natural unrestricted movement allows several degrees of smooth, spontaneous, rotating motion encompassed by the horizontal and vertical planes as long as the bones involved are free to return to rest in neutral, a hub of converging forces that serves as a regulating mechanism. There's nothing wrong with rotation; in an emergency we may need extra flexibility to avoid stumbling or to jump out of harm's way. Incomplete rotation–frozen, stuck, jammed rotation that never returns to neutral and thereby prevents muscles from resetting for repeated contractions–is what's happening. The issue isn't the rotation, per se–your maneuverability depends on it–but rather the inability of the muscles supported by the joints to go home to their starting point where the bones of the hips and shoulders (connected via the spine and working in close conjunction with the knees, ankles and feet) are in vertical and horizontal alignment and close coordination.

Skeptics are always rotated; usually right to left so that the heart is pulled back with the right shoulder and side interposed toward the front. As I pointed out in *The Egoscue Method of Health through Motion,* you can see the rotation in the mirror. One shoulder or hip looks closer than the other. If there is shoulder or hip rotation (or both, which is not at all unusual) your posture is off-balance.

Repeat after me–*the body is a unit.* It is an important mantra.

Everything is connected to everything else. If your shoulders are rotated, that affects your spine, the spine affects your head, the head's position affects vision, balance, hearing, and neural functions. And that's just for openers–rotated shoulders have an impact on the low back and the hips too. The hips are in close collaboration with the knees, the ankles and feet.

In the name of guarding the heart, the skeptic is causing lots of collateral damage. And it does no good to merely point that out. He or she is so distrustful that the information about rotation will be shrugged off as another hypothesis: *You tell me it is rotation; the doctor says it's a bad disk in the spine. I don't know what to believe.*

So the skeptic simply doubts on.

I used to rely on the pain on/pain off approach. I thought that turning off the pain by eliminating the rotation would convince a client that the restoration of postural balance was the cure he or she sought. I didn't understand that skeptics' need to protect the heart took precedence. Their fear of being deceived, tripped up, and trapped blocked awareness. They stayed with their story unless I gave them time and encouragement to realize that by being fully balanced there was no danger that they couldn't face head-on and surmount.

I set out to create a non-threatening atmosphere that allows the feel of balance to slowly emerge from the welter of distractions that hide the facts. And it feels good, very good. Without undergoing the humiliation and fear of losing the security of their story, they gradually wean themselves away from the need for the story and accept the reality that if they are balanced, the heart–as pump and spiritual cornerstone–is invulnerable. By becoming balanced, plugging back into the universal power grid, re-energizing, being present in the moment by not reliving the past or *preliving* the future, they gain peace of mind. Little by little, without needing me to persuade them, the skeptic finally becomes aware that they are enough. They've got energy, strength, calmness, gratitude and great joy. How do they know? They feel it.

Know thyself. Are you a skeptic?
No?

- Have you been saying, "bullshit, bullshit, bullshit" throughout this chapter?
- You're no cynic, right; just a contrarian.
- You've already sampled some of the E-cises and don't think they seem very effective.
- You bought one of my other books and your back, knee, shoulder, whatever still hurts ... this book is more of the same old, same old.
- Is life ugly, brutish and short?
- Are you an optimist or a pessimist? A little of both? Or don't you know?
- Is your body letting you down? Or are you letting your body down? Or are those stupid questions?
- Is it too late?
- How old are you? Does it matter?
- What's your story?
- What do you believe in?
- Are you alone?
- What hurts? Why?
- Have you looked at yourself in the mirror lately? The whole you, not just your face? What did you see? Did you like what you saw? What are you doing about it?
- How do you feel? Why?

Take a long, leisurely walk. Think about those questions and answer two or three of them. By the time you get back home, decide if you are a skeptic. If you are, do the E-cises that conclude this chapter.

If you decide that you are not a skeptic—and that is entirely possible—go on to the next chapter.

E-cise Menu for Skeptics

Foot Circles/Point Flexes

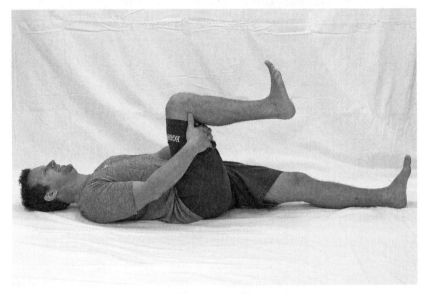

Figure 11-E4

This E-cise restores ankle flexibility and strengthens the flexion and extension muscles. For Foot Circles, lie on your back with one leg extended flat on the floor and the other bent toward the chest. Clasp your hands behind the bent knee while you circle the foot clockwise twenty times. Meanwhile, keep the other leg on the floor with toes pointing straight toward the ceiling. Reverse direction of the circling foot and repeat. Change sides and repeat. Make sure the knee stays absolutely still, with the movement coming from the ankle, not the knee.

For Point Flexes, stay in the same position on your back with one leg extended and the other bent. Bring the toes of the extended leg toward the shin to flex the foot then reverse the direction to point the foot. Twenty flex/point combos, and repeat with the other foot for another twenty (forty total).

Sitting Femur Rotations

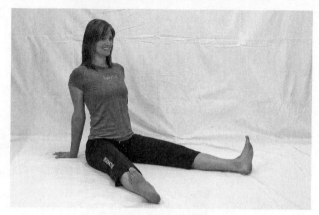

Figure 11-E16 (a)

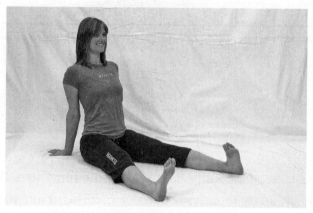

Figure 11-E17 (b)

This E-cise introduces full lateral movement of the knee and ankle via the hip socket. Sit on the floor with both legs extended straight in front of you. Your feet should be eight to ten inches apart. For support, place your hands behind your hips by about four inches. Tighten your thigh muscles, flex your toes, and roll your hips forward to arch your back. Using your hip sockets, rotate your knees and feet inward and then outward. It is important to keep your hips rolled forward, thighs flexed and toes flexed. Do not lean back too heavily on your hands; try to sit up straight with your head and shoulders back. Do three sets of twenty repetitions. (One rotation in and one out count as one.)

Crocodile Twist

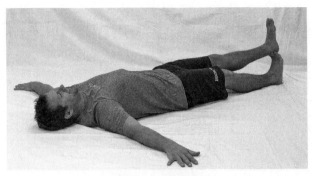

Figure 11-E9 (a)

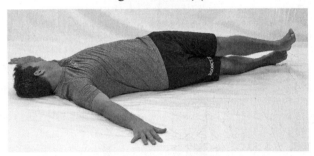

Figure 11-E10 (b)

This E-cise promotes bilateral activity by wringing out the posture muscles of the spine and the hip, making them contract and release equally on both sides—something they have forgotten how to do because of upper torso rotation. Lie on your back with legs extended flat on the floor. Point the toes of your right foot at the ceiling, heel on the floor. Put the heel of your left foot on the toes of your right foot (the right big toe will be the primary contact point). Extend your arms to the side, level with the shoulders, palms facing the floor. Tighten the thigh muscles (quadriceps) of both legs and roll your feet to the right, getting them to touch the floor, while keeping one foot aligned atop the other. As you do this, lift your left hip off the floor, pointing it at the ceiling. Your head looks to the left (get your ear as close to the floor as possible). Hold this position and breathe; keep the thighs tight. Reverse the feet and repeat on the other side. One minute on each side.

Cats & Dogs

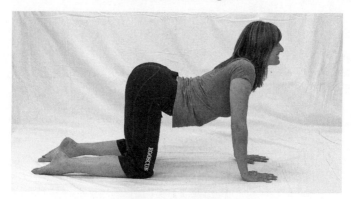

Figure 11-E11 (a)

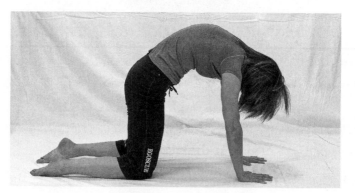

Figure 11-E12 (b)

This E-cise works the hips, spine, shoulders and neck in coordinated flexion-extension. Get down on the floor on your hands and knees. Make sure your knees are aligned with your hips, your wrists and your shoulders; your lower legs should be parallel with each other and with your hips. Make sure your weight is distributed evenly. Smoothly round your back as your head curls under to create a curve that runs from the buttocks to the neck—this is the cat with an arched back. Smoothly sway the back down while bringing the head up—now the perky dog. Make these two moves flow continuously back and forth rather than allowing them to be distinct and choppy. Do ten repetitions.

Standing at Wall with Pillow between Knees

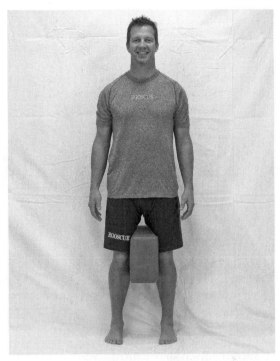

Figure 11-E29

This E-cise promotes proper positioning of all load joints with the wall as the template. Stand at a wall with your feet parallel and hips-width apart. Your heels, hips, upper back and *maybe* your head are against a wall. *Maybe* because some people have severe shoulder rotation and/or slumping which pull the neck and head forward. If so, bring your head up and back toward the wall as far as it will go without forcing it. Over time as you do this E-cise the muscles will gradually strengthen enough to bring the back of your head into contact with the wall. Relax your stomach muscles and make sure that your feet remain pointed straight ahead. An inflatable small pillow between your knees should feel as if it is slightly pushing the knees apart. Do not push into the pillow; it is there to trigger some of your hip muscles to provide stabilization while you are in this position. Hold for four minutes.

Static Extension Position

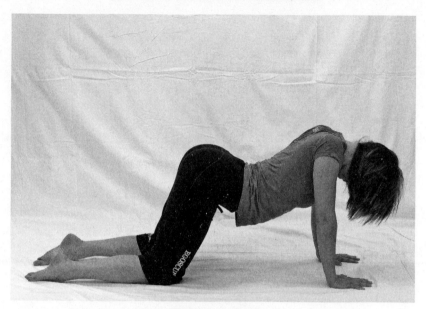

Figure 11-E13

This E-cise counteracts hip rotation. Start on your hands and knees on the floor. Move your hands forward by about six inches, then move your upper body forward so that your shoulders are above your hands. Your hips are now in front of your knees by about six inches. Keep your elbows straight, and allow your shoulder blades to collapse together while your low back arches. It arches because your hips roll forward, allowing the movement to occur. Drop your head. Stay in this position for three minutes.

Sitting Knee Pillow Squeezes

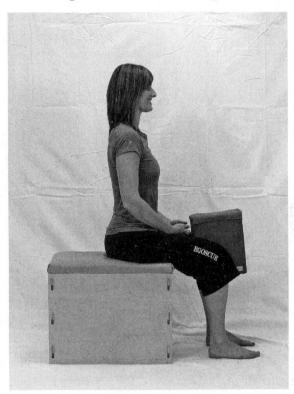

Figure 11-E18

This E-cise promotes bilateral pelvic extension and encourages pelvic stability. Sit toward the front edge of a hard chair (don't lean into the chair back) with a thick pillow or inflatable block between your knees, your pelvis rolled forward to put an arch in your lower back. Keep your feet pointed straight ahead and your upper body relaxed. Squeeze and release the pillow between your knees; keep the arch in your low back. Remember, your feet are pointed straight ahead. Three sets of twenty repetitions each.

Sitting Abductor Press with Strap

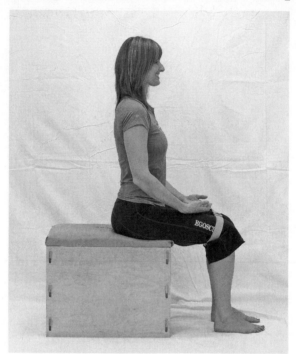

Figure 11-E19

This E-cise develops bilateral pelvic extension and encourages pelvic stability. Sit in a chair with your feet pointed straight ahead. A four-foot-long, non-elastic strap with a buckle is needed for this E-cise (or you can improvise with an old belt or a length of rope). Buckle or tie the strap around your knees, with your knees hips-width apart. Roll your pelvis forward to place a small arch into your lower back. Do not lean back. As you hold this low-back arch, which was hip-induced, push outward against the strap at your knees and release. Do three sets for twenty repetitions each.

Standing Arm Circles, Palms Down
with Pillow between Knees

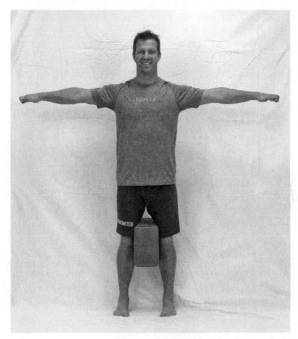

Figure 11-E24

This E-cise promotes bilateral lumbar function through thoracic stabilization. Stand facing a full-length mirror with your
feet pointed straight ahead, a pillow or inflatable block between your knees. Place your finger tips into the pad of each
hand and point your thumbs straight out. This hand position is
imperative to the exercise being done correctly. It is called the
"golfer's grip." Squeeze your shoulder blades together and
bring your arms out to your sides at shoulder level. With your
palms facing downward and thumbs straight ahead, circle up
and forward for one hundred repetitions. With your palms facing upward, circle up and back for another one hundred repetitions. Remember to keep your feet straight and your shoulder
blades squeezed together.

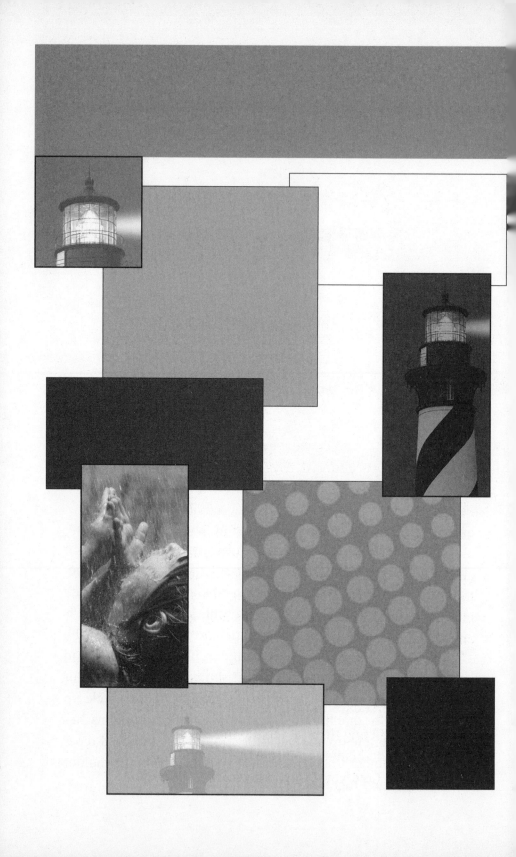

CHAPTER

12

Making the Worst of It

Of the three predominant AAE pattern personality types, pessimists don't just tell their story—they are their story. Cynics like to proclaim that "life is just one damned thing after another." I couldn't disagree more, but pessimists are certain that they live under an unrelenting siege. Their story collects the damned things of their life and bolts the fragments together into an intricate narrative that serves both as a script and as an alibi:

- How bad things keep happening to a good person
- Why the worst case trumps the best of intentions
- And the addicting thrill of identifying the one who bears the blame for all the pain, limitation and despair (and you can guess who the Who is)

Yes, it gets pretty gnarly. A pessimist's story is a litany of woe that spreads incident by incident, event by event, and typically covers ten to twenty years of soap opera-like plot development in which boundless hope, the most powerful medicine of all, gives way to oppressive negativity. But that's no soap opera—it's the stuff of personal tragedy and searing emotional pain.

No, I should have known better.

No, that was a mistake.

No … I'm afraid it's too late.

Pessimists are willing to take long treks into the distant past to relive accidents, illnesses, disappointments and assorted mishaps. They pass harsh judgment on themselves, wallow in recriminations, and fulminate at the injustice. Their stories are epic and comprehensive; great heaps of rubble that block the way and keep the narrator-protagonist from either moving forward to a fresh start or toward taking responsibility for their own history and health.

Pessimists can recover their positive energy flow, peace of mind and perfect health only by putting down the burden of their story, by reopening a connection to the present. It's not easy. But you can do it. You are enough.

When I was a young Marine second lieutenant in Vietnam, my commanding officer got fed up with the indecision I was demonstrating during a firefight—it was my first time leading troops in combat, and I was dithering back and forth between options as I conferred with him on the field radio. He barked at me, "Make up your mind, Lieutenant … don't die wondering." Good advice. So stop wondering, assume you are one of the pessimists and do something about it.

In the clinic, we help pessimists put down their burdensome stories by reintroducing postural balance, which always calms the mind and restores the flow of positive energy. Since you've already read the chapters about fact collectors and skeptics, you are probably not surprised to wind up back here in the weeds of postural therapy. There's one big difference, though: this is the intensive care ward. If I were forced to do triage—and, fortunately, I'm not—I would turn away the fact collectors and the skeptics and work only with the pessimists. They are in the deepest trouble.

The story is literally eating them alive. It is blocking the high wavelength energy needed to maintain health and sustain a pain-free, satisfying life.

The pessimists are my biggest worry. They are dying. I'm immediately tempted to go on the attack and rip up the story. But that would make things worse. Without at least restoring the tiniest bit of balance first, a frontal assault on the story will fail. Usually someone living in a bubble of pessimism gets offended by the suggestion that he is to blame (even though no such implication was intended). The story, while deeply disturbing, is familiar, comforting; it's a security blanket and, rather than give it up, he backs off, loses interest in the Method as postural therapy, makes excuses, or starts arguing. Perversely, he is proud of his story, fiercely protective of it. After all, he is at the center of the tale, heroically enduring outrageous slings and arrows. The story amounts to a "green card" that, instead of attesting to citizenship, signifies that the bearer tried his best to write a happy ending to the story and now it is up to someone else.

The pessimists are the divas of show-and-tell. Their story is on a conversational loop that plays and replays. Even so, I'm willing to listen to a story over and over again, waiting for an opportunity to ask, "What would you like to do now?"

Parsing Pronouns

A word or two about gender and pronouns: As I have for Fact Collectors and Skeptics, I am switching genders to establish that these personality types are common in both men and women. There was a time when an author could just use "he," "him," and "his," but not anymore. If an example seems to reflect a gender stereotype given my choice of pronoun, simply plug in another pronoun more to your liking; they are totally interchangeable.

Often, the answer is something like, "I just don't know. They've tried everything."

"You told me that your neck hurts—nine-and-a-half on a ten-point scale. Since you are here today, do you think it makes sense to see if we can knock that down a little, say to a six or seven, if we can?"

"I don't know. You can try."

Cue the fireworks, the balloon drop, and confetti. In the initial phase of working with the pessimist, "I don't know. You can try ..." is as good as it gets. He doesn't have the energy to invest in even low-grade enthusiasm. He is running on empty. The remarkable thing is that he is even running at all. Pessimists are nearly helpless but they are most helpful and, miraculously, still hopeful. Their stories have blotted out every survival instinct except one last trace of hope. Instead of quitting, they hang on to a last vestige of against-the-odds belief—belief, not in themselves, but in the experts whom they have turned to for aid. This is a mixed blessing, but if that's what we've got to work with—so be it.

High Hopes

When a pessimist first arrives at one of our clinics, she is certain we will rescue her from pain. T.N. was a good example. She had researched the Egoscue Method and was convinced it was the silver bullet. Yet that certainty was undermined by her conviction that she would screw it up. Why? Her story proved it. Time and time again, she had consulted the best minds of medicine and health care, main-stream, experimental and alternative practitioners who have stellar reputations and solid track records. She followed their advice, underwent unpleasant treatments and dutifully sub-mitted to expensive tests, patronizing lectures, and intrusive examinations. It was typical. Undaunted on the surface, our pessimist friend kept at it, but the only things to show for the effort were more pain, less energy and another chapter to her story about a woman who tried and failed. There is no way to argue the pessimist out of this poisonous mindset. She lis-tened intently, nodded gravely and said, "What you're saying has merit, but I just don't know."

And how right she was! She didn't know. Thinking her way out is not on. She must feel her way to positive expecta-tions that can serve as the fulcrum for action. By gently nudg-ing the pessimist toward a decision to take action based on what she feels, and by framing it in low-key terms, I leave the story in place without directly disputing the failure expecta-tion that provides its foundation. It is more effective to offer unconditional support and signal that I accept her as a good person who is willing to keep trying even though the effort may not lead to dramatic progress (or any progress at all). Al-though I personally expect improvement, I don't openly chal-lenge her self-defeating story because that would provoke a stubborn defense that usually leaves the pessimist opting to go elsewhere for help rather than give up her story. If I want her to stick with me and decide to take the next step, it cannot be my choice. Typically, experts relieve the non-expert of the need to make decisions. This is true of plumbing experts, fi-nancial experts, medical experts, experts of all sorts. Experts are professionally and emotionally invested in a treatment methodology, stand ready and eager to implement it, and as-sume—not at all unreasonably—that that is precisely why they are being consulted.

> **Unawareness**
> Meditation and other techniques provide a means of conscious access to and the awareness of actuating beliefs. Emotional turmoil is a consequence of one's inability to achieve an enlightened awareness.

In reality, pessimists want experts to validate their story and cure the problem, but that's impossible. Why? Human health is influenced by what I call *actuating belief*. If I take over, it means removing the actuating belief that was part of her original physiological equipment and replacing it with the belief that I'm in charge of her health. She must believe that she is a passive bystander. Total buy-in is required. To do that, however, the expert must repeal Existential Health Law # 1:

Healing and health come from within the individual.

Passive bystanders and experts are outsiders by definition. Hence, a pessimist only thinks she believes that the expert is the answer to her prayers. What she actually believes is just the opposite. Her aware mind, not the thinking mind, instinctively embraces all the fundamental realities of existence because they actuate existence itself, thereby becoming forms of unalterable transcendent belief. An individual may not be enlightened enough to be consciously aware of an actuating belief, but his or her physiological systems are fully attuned. That's not to say that actuating beliefs shield us from the folly of our thinking minds or our inability to fully access the aware mind. The unaware, the unenlightened, pay a high price. They persist in taking actions (thoughts are both forms of action and forms of matter/energy) that undermine their health and well-being by diverting and draining off positive, high wavelength energy.

By deferring to experts and handing over to them personal responsibility for her health, the pessimist loses important benefits that would otherwise reach her by way of the actuating and actionable belief that health comes from within. She is closing down a vital feedback loop that provides energy, strength and confidence. If this happened only occasionally or temporarily, it wouldn't be a big deal. The human body has a genius for problem-solving and coping with the unexpected, but when experts take charge by orchestrating onslaughts of toxic chemical compounds and traumatic surgical intervention, on top of a modern culture that features poor nutritional standards and acutely sedentary lifestyles, the cumulative damage can be enormous and lasting.

It is not possible to simultaneously believe and disbelieve, which is what the pessimist attempts to do. As powerful as the thinking mind is, it cannot erase existential belief derived from biological reality. Thoughts are things. The thought—confirmed by the experience of allowing the expert to usurp power—delivers the message *you are not enough*, and that attitude suppresses healing when a pessimist is chased away from her rightful, paramount role as the primary health generator and guardian. That's what I mean when I use the term *actuating belief*. By believing in the expert and disbelieving her own power, she ends up losing the very thing she depends on to guarantee health and well-being.

Belief is the mind's thumb. Like the thumbs of our hands, which allow us the flexibility, control, strength and delicate touch to make and grasp tools, belief gives us the power to use the mind in a deliberate and structured way. It links thought to action. If you do not believe there are fish in the pond, you won't go fishing. Indeed, the practical effect is the same no matter what the actual conditions—no fish. If you don't believe that the aspirin will get rid of your headache, it probably won't. If you believe the chemotherapy will kill you before it cures your cancer, it probably will.

Belief can serve as an on-off switch that activates or deactivates important supporting physiological mechanisms. Notice that I said *supporting*. Medical treatment isn't magic; mostly it is chemistry or, in the case of surgery, sophisticated forms of carpentry and plumbing. Hit living tissue with a hammer and it reacts, but after that happens, then what? Physical discomfort, pain and health in general are extremely subjective states. Our senses receive stimuli that lack a uniform objective basis because sensory perception is unique to the individual. Humans raise physical sensation to the level of perception by assigning meaning and value to a biochemical and neurological event that involves impingement on receptor cells of a sensory organ such as the eye, ear or skin, as well as a vast range of sensory mechanisms that are only now beginning to be fully appreciated by cutting-edge science.

By transferring responsibility to the expert, a pessimist sits back and waits to feel a positive or negative sensation. And waits and waits and waits. Deep down, he really expects the negative. What he thinks he believes in, usually half heartedly—the expert's educational credentials and state-of-the-art tools—are unlikely to produce a sensation capable of overcoming the pervasive fear that is blocking the flow of positive energy he needs to regain health. The body's internal scanning mechanism finds only an overactive thinking mind coping with an idea—powerlessness—that is at odds with biological experience.

Am I saying that all medical and expert-managed intervention is ineffective? No. But effectiveness is a direct consequence of the individual's belief system. In the case of the pessimist, that belief system is impaired by an expectation of failure, much of it generated by a story that neatly 'confirms' that a bad outcome is inevitable. Repeated over and over, until the certainty overwhelms awareness of any lingering ingrained remnants of optimism, fallen rose petals on the verge of being whirled away by a sudden storm. Successes that occur are a result of treatment that happens to get under the radar of those expectations, principally by triggering deep-seated unconscious beliefs (and their supporting positive emotions) which manage to operate independently of the failure expectations and counteract their deadly effects.

Access to the aware mind is of great importance. By putting the pessimist back in charge of her expectations and her health through reestablishing postural balance, it is possible to place her at the center of things, where she can decide to take up her responsibilities instead of handing them off to outsiders. Restoration of postural balance won't happen all at once, and may not happen at all. Even so, it is essential to try to move in the right direction, to encourage the pessimist to resume taking small portions of responsibility, which can be gradually expanded. It is a way to slowly regain lost confidence, ratchet down the sense of helplessness, muzzle the fear of powerlessness and begin to rebuild the capacity to absorb positive energy.

You can feel it! You'll know when it's time to drop that story.

Pessimists have lost their aware minds. The obsession with story blocks awareness by leading them back into the past and/or ahead into the future (usually both). Only the present is energized, however. Every moment that the mind spends outside of the present by rehashing events and situations that no longer exist as a way to *learn from mistakes*–which is really an excuse to find fault with one's self–is a moment disconnected from the universal energy grid. Similarly, imagining future events that will never take place, except possibly in the roughest approximation, also cuts her off from the supply of high wavelength energy. Pessimists are in the habit of reliving the past and preliving the future. Consequently, they are in an acute state of energy deprivation.

Their despair is palpable. In *The Egoscue Method of Health through Motion* I described Condition III's as having the posture of despair: hips tilted under as though a pair of hands had gripped them from behind and yanked them forward and down with tremendous force, flattening the S-curve of the spine (the "S" is actually reversed – like this – Ƨ) so that when the pelvis tilts under, the lower curve no longer bellies to the left (which is what gives us spinal strength, balance and flexibility), sending the shoulders forward, rounded and slumped, and leaving the head to jut forward. It is the signature posture of the pessimist. Stiff and unbalanced, she struggles to stay upright as gravity seeks to topple her to the earth face-first. Her shoulders and knees torque and wobble to keep her moving forward in a straight line. She trips and falls frequently. Walking is stressful, climbing stairs agonizing, and running rips up joints and courts a heart attack. Their lifestyles aren't to blame, heredity has little to do with it, and there's nothing wrong with the design of their body. This looks like energy starvation—and it *is* energy starvation. The pessimist is very familiar. She looks like your neighbor, your daughter, your boss. Glance in the mirror; she may look like you.

When asked how they feel right now, the question is always a show-stopper. Pessimists don't have the vocabulary handy to describe the present moment so they launch into a report on what their physician believes is wrong, the latest side effects of the medicine, and the headaches that interfere with their resolutions to get more exercise and a good night's sleep. These stories are layered with symptoms, tests, mistakes, and unforeseen complications.

I'll respond: "No, that's how you felt last week when you went to see the doctor. How do you feel right now?"

"The same."

"Tell me how the 'same' feels."

"It hurts."

"Where?"

Pessimists seem almost reluctant to pinpoint the pain. The reason is that a specific locus of pain has morphed and diffused into a general sensation that is part pain, part fear, part metabolic slowdown and part physiological exhaustion. Pessimists are being flooded with incomings calls from their internal sensors, warning that their system is sliding into a catastrophic state of deterioration. Actual pain—the I-can't-bend-my-knee-without-screaming kind of pain—is the least of their worries.

Most pessimists have gotten accustomed to feeling lousy, but it is impossible to fake a sunny outlook on life. They are glum, anxious and weary. When I ask where it hurts, the idea of being able to focus on a single ache or pain seems strange. It would make more sense to ask where it doesn't hurt. They have come to expect to feel bad, and deal with it by treating their symptoms like cantankerous old friends or beloved pets that must be coddled and indulged; otherwise they'll act up and behave badly. As for the future, they don't anticipate a change for the better.

There is a reverse placebo effect (known as the nocebo effect) that pessimists bring into the offices of health care practitioners of every stripe that makes progress extremely unlikely. If a patient believes the visit will help make him feel better, he will actually show signs of improvement a day or so before the visit takes place: a classic placebo effect.[14] But when the pessimist believes that nothing will help—guess what? Nothing helps. The powers of intention, attention and expectation have enormous effect. Thoughts are things. The body responds to

---

[14] In recent years, the placebo effect has grown more pronounced. The FDA uses sugar pills in trials of new drugs to measure how much benefit is derived from a new drug's ingredients and how much comes from the placebo. Half of all drugs tested are pulled from the testing pipeline because they can't beat the sugar pills. This phenomenon has increased by more than one-third since the 1980s.

the mind by adjusting blood and brain chemistry, altering the permeability of cellular membranes and increasing oxygen flow. A third power, the power of awareness, is at work too. By tuning out the present and focusing instead on her story filled with shadows of the past, a pessimist cannot marshal her full physical and mental resources. In Shakespeare's *Henry IV, Part 1*, the mouthy Welsh warlord Glendower brags that he can win a crucial battle by calling on supernatural powers from the "vasty deep."

"Why, so can I, or so can any man," replies Hotspur, who then asks blandly, "but will they come when you do call?" A pessimist's formidable inner powers may never hear the call to join in today's battle because she is looking toward the past, not the present. As a result, the forces of hope and life do not come to the rescue. Worse, they are actively turned away.[15]

Energy surrounds and saturates all living things like the sea that washes around a coral reef, bathing, nurturing, and healing its teeming efflorescence. The living reef is embraced by the sea's life-giving energy; it opens itself to the current and lives. The embrace is all. As long as the powers of intention, attention, expectation and awareness are switched off or pointed elsewhere, there can be no transfer of energy, no embrace, and soon—no life.

The thrilling thing about pessimists is that they can turn on a dime once they get a little traction. By putting their story aside for as little as ten minutes while they concentrate on a few basic balancing exercises, a rush of incoming energy can blast the pessimist out of the hole she has dug for herself. The present floods in and saturates her with a sense of well-being.

---

[15] Glendower's forces do not rally and the young, noble Hotspur dies on the battlefield.

By encouraging pessimists to take small, simple steps to restore musculoskeletal system balance without tying it to the
story one way or the other (if the story is never heard of again,
good riddance!), a postural therapist can quickly help boost
their metabolism and send their mood soaring. In short order,
the pessimist's story starts losing relevance and power. Within
a very few days, as her postural balance improves, she finds that
her focus has shifted away from her story and onto the present.
Her aware mind blossoms; fear no longer stalks her. She marvels at the enjoyment derived from a short walk to visit friends
and a brisk stroll on the beach at low tide to collect shells,
something she hasn't done for years. You are enough after all.

Come on, give it a try. Embrace the present moment. Always catch the rain.

E-cise Menu for Pessimists

Standing Pigeon-toed at the Wall

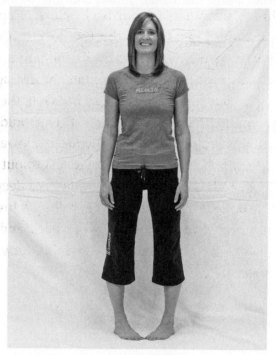

Figure 12-E31 (a)

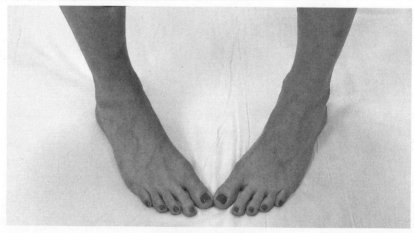

Figure 12-E32 (b)

This E-cise is a wake-up call directed at hip muscles that are snoozing instead of doing their job to smoothly tip the pelvic bowl from a neutral (level) position (side to side and front to back) to one that tips forward as you walk across varied terrain and then return to neutral. Otherwise, you rely on popping your knees and wagging your back, spine, shoulders and head to induce the hip to allow the legs to flex and extend. Stand with your heels, buttocks, back, shoulders and head against the wall. Feel both your shoulder blades against the wall. Make sure the back of your head contacts the wall and that you are not arching your shoulders. Feet should be parallel and about hips-width apart. Swivel your feet inward so that the big toes touch. Keep the angle of the feet about the same during the E-cise. Relax your stomach and take deep breaths. If your head won't stay against the wall, roll up a towel or use an inflatable roll and put it between your neck and the wall. Keep your hands at your sides, thumbs facing forward. Hold for four to six minutes.

Standing Forward Bend

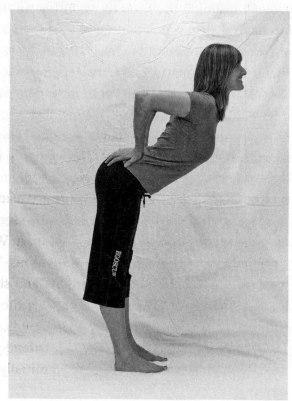

Figure 12-E26

This E-cise loosens the hamstring muscles of the leg that become tight and generally inflexible from disuse and it re-integrates the functions of the hip, lumbar spine, thoracic back and shoulders. Our ancestors didn't have to worry about this because they frequently bent over at the waist and sat on the ground. Place your feet flat on the floor, parallel and about hips-width apart. Put your hands on your hips as if you were going to slide the thumbs into your back pants pockets. The thumbs should point straight down the legs. Slowly lean forward at the waist and while you keep your hands in contact with your hips, draw your elbows back toward each other. Don't flap; slowly pull them back as your back descends and you lift your head. Keep your back flat; don't arch it. What you are doing is reintegrating your upper torso functions. They are designed to work together. Find a comfortable and stable position as far forward as you can without arching the back or letting the shoulders sag. Hold this for thirty seconds. You will gradually become more limber and be able to extend your upper torso well beyond what you were able to initially achieve the first couple of times.

In-line Gluteal Contractions

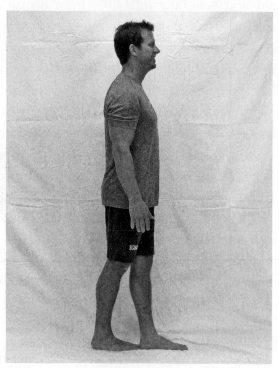

Figure 12-E27

This E-cise reminds your glute muscles (*musculus gluteus*) in each buttock that they don't just sit around. Among other functions, they handle the proper movement of the feet, keep the pelvis from tipping forward, and allow leg extension for stair-climbing. Stand with the heel of your left foot touching the tips of your right toes. The feet will be flat on the floor and in a straight line. Knees locked. Balance your hips evenly to the right and left (they may want to rotate and swing your torso around) by equalizing your weight on both feet and keeping your head and shoulders back. Simultaneously contract and release both the right and left glutes. Do three sets of twenty. Switch the feet (left in front of right), contract and release the glutes for another three sets of twenty. Don't use your abdominal muscles. Make the contractions full, smooth and slow. If you have trouble retaining your balance, use a chair or a wall for support.

Static Extension Position

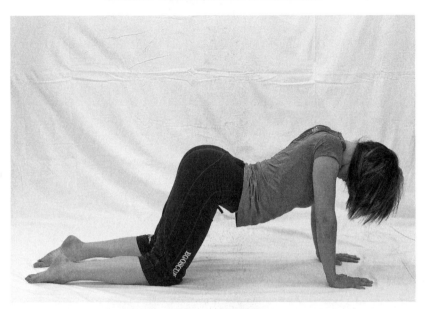

Figure 12-E13

This E-cise counteracts hip rotation. Start on your hands and knees on the floor. Move your hands forward by about six inches, then move your upper body forward so that your shoulders are above your hands. Your hips are now in front of your knees by about six inches. Keep your elbows straight, and allow your shoulder blades to collapse together while your low back arches. It arches because your hips roll forward, allowing the movement to occur. Drop your head. Stay in this position for three minutes.

Cats & Dogs

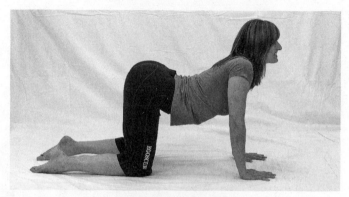

Figure 12-E11 (a)

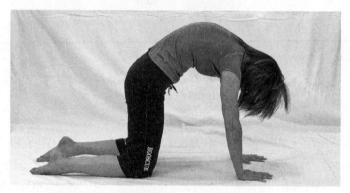

Figure 12-E12 (b)

This E-cise works the hips, spine, shoulders and neck in coordinated flexion-extension. Get down on the floor on your hands and knees. Make sure your knees are aligned with your hips, your wrists and your shoulders. Your lower legs should be parallel with each other and with your hips. Make sure your weight is distributed evenly. Smoothly round your back as your head curls under to create a curve that runs from the buttocks to the neck—this is the cat with an arched back. Smoothly sway the back down while bringing the head up—now the perky dog. Make these two moves flow continuously back and forth rather than allowing them to be distinct and choppy. Ten repetitions (one cat plus one dog count as one).

Downward Dog

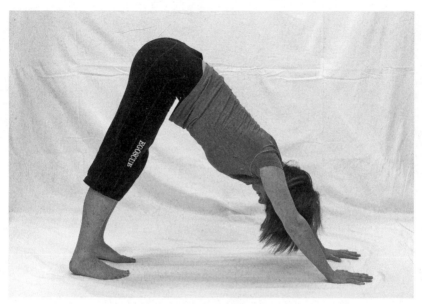

Figure 12-E14

This E-cise reestablishes linkage from the wrists to the feet. Assume the Cats & Dogs starting position (see above). Curl your toes under, and push with your legs to raise your torso until you are off your knees with the weight resting on your hands and feet. Keep pushing until your hips are higher than your shoulders and have formed a tight, stable triangle with the floor. Your knees should be straight, your calves and thighs tight. Don't let your feet flair outward; keep them pointing straight ahead in line with your hands, which need to stay in place–no creeping backward. Your back should be flat, not bowed, as you hips press up and back into the heels. Breathe. If you cannot bring your heels flat onto the floor, get them as close as possible. Don't force them. It may take several sessions before they go all the way down. Remain in this position for one minute.

Towel-rolls Settle (with a strap)

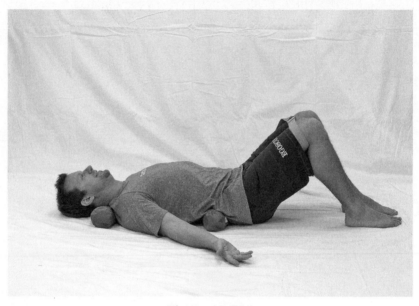

Figure 12-E15

This E-cise allows gravity to relax and release the muscles of the upper body. You'll need two bath towels folded in half and rolled. Lie on your back with knees bent and held together with a belt or non-elastic strap. Your feet should be flat on the floor and placed parallel about hips-width apart. Place one of the rolled towels under the back of your neck (don't rest your head on it; it is there to support your neck) and the other goes under your low back and just above the hips. Hold this position for ten minutes.

Cats & Dogs Redux

See Figure 12-E11 (a), Figure 12-E12 (b) on page 162.

See the instructions and illustrations above. Don't rush through these; take your time and enjoy them.

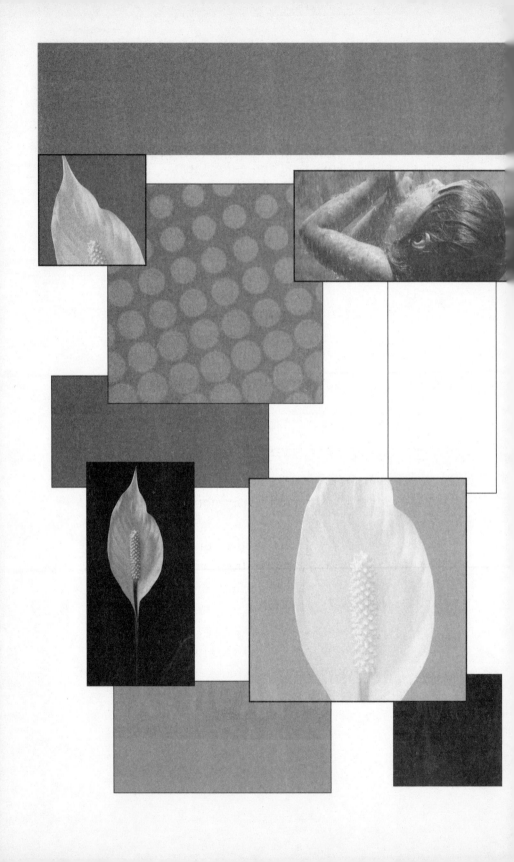

Unstick This

Okay. The Big Three.

You're up, it's time to make a decision and take action.

Sonya, a well-known Hollywood actor, faced the same challenge after making only three visits to my San Diego clinic. She was hesitating and when I asked her what she wanted to do, immediately replied, "Whatever you say."

I guess we know where she was coming from—straight from Planet Pessimism. What I said to her also applies to you, no matter where you are coming from: "Why not go with whatever the body says?"

Fortunately, he or she who hesitates is not lost, just bogged down. Start getting unstuck right here by answering a couple of easy questions: *How do you feel after doing each of the E-cise menus that I introduced in Chapters 10 11 and 12? What's happening physically and emotionally when you read them over and—most important—when you tried them?* Focus. You've just finished stimulating what amounts to the most sensitive, hyper-responsive life form that has ever existed. From the soles of your feet to the top of your skull there was (and still is) an uproar of signals, enzyme releases, hormone drips, adjustments and status reports. More than 100 million protein molecules per cell are being concocted, dissolved and reassembled at any given instant. It is absurd to think that such an intricate, hair-trigger device just sits there dead in the water.

My firm belief is that the aware mind is capable of dialing in to any single cell in the body to receive a precisely detailed readout of the weather that is occurring within the ecosystems that are encompassed by the cellular membranes of all 60 trillion grains of life. Yes, you can fine-tune your awareness to listen in on all this and infinitely more. Even if you are dealing with a serious chronic illness, the content of the message traffic is overwhelmingly positive. Only a tiny fraction of the content is reporting anomalies. Our earliest ancestors joyfully belly-flopped into the torrent of positive data and were carried for tens of thousands of years straight into adventures that drove other seemingly superior life-forms into extinction. Sadly, as of late, the trip has taken us on a detour from brash self-confidence to the doorstep of self-loathing. But we are in the process of getting back on the main highway.

And your decision is…?

Oh, you haven't done the E-cises yet. (If you have—good! Skip the next paragraph as your reward.)

I have been taking it easy, maybe too easy, on giving a lot of explicit instructions in each chapter because I want you to call the shots. This isn't a cookbook that you can flip through, read a recipe, imagine how good it tastes and turn to the next recipe and the next. I use the term "menu" for a reason. For one thing, "routine" and "program" make it sound like drudgery. The allusion to eating is apt because you need to get the benefits of these E-cises into your system. If you don't actually sample the items on the menus you are letting your thinking mind control the play. This is where your story starts getting in the way. A fact collector is probably thinking, "I need more facts." The skeptic concludes, "It can't be that simple." And the pessimists hide out in their steadily shrinking comfort zones, muttering, "I can't do this myself." The plot always thickens. It is the reason our stories grow so large and cumbersome that eventually we are unable to move forward.

We all experience occasional brief bouts of indecision. However, chronic indecision is a symptom of a serious energy deficit. It takes a huge supply of energy to make important decisions and carry them out promptly, particularly those with many moving parts and potential complications. Individuals who are balanced, aware and at peace with themselves can effortlessly draw on their abundant energy resources. Hence, decision-making is no big deal. Any energy they use is promptly replaced. In contrast, when the fuel gauge is stuck on low, the tendency is to cut back on consumption; even small decisions seem enormous. When the energy shortage is prolonged—*those who are shackled to one of the three archetypal stories*—the body is forced to retreat into the thinking mind which substitutes various dodges like *wait-and-see, pass the buck* or cynicism because other options requiring action further deplete the already inadequate amount of energy that remains available.

What we are trying to do is get you out of your thinking mind long enough to jumpstart the flow of positive energy. You don't have to go into the E-cises cold; do a short series of prefatory warm-ups:

- Stand with your weight evenly distributed on each foot, eyes closed
- Inhale and exhale deeply and slowly to a count of thirty
- Listen to the sounds inside and outside the room
- Imagine that you are looking down on yourself from above
- Be grateful for the moment

An important thing is taking place during these preliminaries: I am sneaking you extra energy, just enough to clear away the fog and engage your feeling mind. In addition, each item on the menu itself will supply a small spurt of energy as it restores (a little) postural alignment and balance.

One of these three menus will prompt your body to speak up louder and clearer than the others because the E-cises and their sequencing are having more impact on your musculoskeletal system's dysfunctions and misalignment. What's more, they are also getting through to your emotions and beginning to calm your mind. I suggest you try one—start with any of the three—and complete a different full menu each day for three days. On the third day, stand in a balanced position with your eyes closed, count slowly to thirty focusing on your breathing, and then, without pondering, chose. Just chose; don't try to explain, weigh, grade or justify. Go with the menu that feels right. What do I mean by "right"?

That's a question I can't answer for you. You'll know it when you feel it.

Do that menu once a day for ten days. After each daily session, spend four or five minutes quietly listening to your body.

Deliberately focus your attention on areas where there is pain, restriction or limitation. It is not necessary to judge, evaluate or compare; just become aware of the available sensations. Use this time to celebrate your body's many gifts.

The simple act of appreciation, of gratitude, can change the interior climate of the body from stressful to blissful. It is an antidote to the waves of fear that can roil the body and wreak havoc with the finely calibrated processes when we lose faith in our perfection. Pain is not an enemy. You have no enemies within unless you open the gates and invite them in.

Gate-keeping is one of your body's most important functions. The membrane of each cell admits only carefully screened, beneficial material—that which has been signed, sealed and delivered by evolution—while denying access to everything else. Cell biologist Dr. Bruce Lipton's brilliant research shows that the cell membrane scrutinizes the incoming matter in search of a key. When found, it activates the formation of a corresponding keyhole and lock mechanism (a necklace-like string of amino acids comprising a protein chain). The key opens a channel into the cell only if there is an exact match of key and keyhole. In other words, sustaining the cell with food, fuel and other essentials is the work of the vigilant membrane—not DNA. The gate-keeper closes the border when it detects danger. Hence, slight changes in valance, pH, turbidity, resonance and a host of other subtle characteristics can lead to a protective cell lockdown.

Fear sends out powerful neurotransmitters that lead to the equivalent of a code-red alert. Apparently even imaginary fears, pessimism, doubts, habitual negativity and anxiety can lead to partial or all-out restrictions in cellular access since such emotions may be legitimate symptoms of disease. The environment outside the cells, therefore, affects the environment within the cells. Blockading the re-supply route into the cells, even if it is only a fraction of the entire sixty trillion, creates negative capability. Fundamentally, all actions are an expression of belief. Our beliefs—life is essentially good versus life is ugly, brutish and short—essentially control our health by allowing expectation to express or distort perception. Bruce Lipton refers to it as "The Biology of Belief." He is exactly right.

Biologists use electron microscopes to discern cell behavior on this level; I contend that all you need is a mirror. In it is visible the tangible, physical expression of the biology of belief in the form of functional posture. If action is an expression of belief, posture is an expression of action(s). By way of original intent, posture's purpose is to effectuate common, everyday actions and fundamental belief—walking, running, throwing, stretching, embracing a mate, cuddling a child, striking an enemy, giving a gift to a friend, and so on—all expressions of fundamental belief in the wisdom of the body. One quick look at our posture tells us what we are capable or incapable of doing.

Glancing in the mirror—literally and figuratively, since we need no looking-glass to truly know our posture—the perception processes of the body provide feedback on who we are and who we can be; our confidence ebbs and flows; energy levels adjust. Best of all, posture is what-you-see-is-what-you-get: It provides an honest template of enormous potential and awesome nobility.

These E-cises have the power to switch postural awareness back on. You will feel the body responding to the stimulus and informing you about what is working and what isn't. Be patient. Expect success. If you are still uncertain, don't force it. Take a day or two off and then try again. As you run through the menu, note any changes: Is an E-cise harder than the last time? Easier?

Give the menu another full ten days. Meanwhile, bump up your physical activity levels. Go for a walk, work in the garden, dance. Monitor your moods, sleep and appetite.

You should feel changes. If not, run through the same series of steps with the other menus.

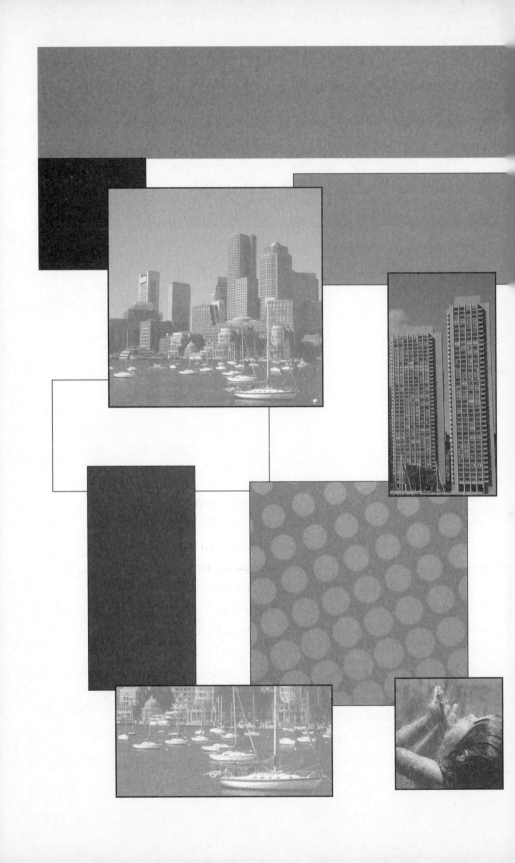

Wall to Wall, Y'all

I would be hugely disappointed if this conversation of ours ended in a thick fog of words. To avoid the danger, I will invoke the Less Is More Rule by turning to a classic technique for achieving brevity and clarity: the Chinese wall poster (my version).

First, an important adjuration (now there's one from the thesaurus ...). Less is more when it comes to cool 1950-ish Studebakers, Barcelona chairs or Bauhaus-inspired office buildings. More is more when you are soaking up positive energy, balance, awareness and motion. It is impossible to overindulge in the items on this menu. For every one of my wall posters add two or three or thirty of your own. Crank up the positive vibes. Go for it.

The human body teaches those who pay attention to put cynicism aside.

If something seems too good to be true, it probably is true.

A symptom is part of a process, not an event.

Change is not something to do. You must allow change.

Allow change from the heart and your head will follow.

Suffering Is Optional.

You are Not Broken.

Ask Why.

Don't keep score, have fun.

Negative thoughts are the single worst health habit.

It is never as bad as you think.

A path without obstacles has no destination.

You are pretty smart. But your body is smarter.

A health expert – any health expert – cannot tell you anything you don't already know.

Never fear Yourself.

Pain is the body's voice. Listen To Your Body.

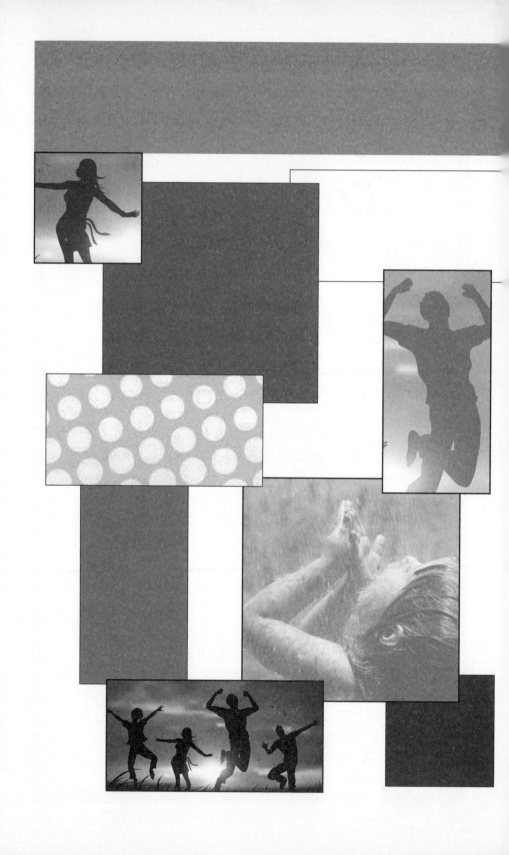

Conclusion

Some authors end a book with a carefully composed overview or they offer up an inspirational peroration to motivate the reader to apply the lessons they have learned.

But I'm going to rewind to Chapter 2 and push "play."

Take off your shoes and socks.

And stand up. Please.

If you are driving a car and listening (I hope you're not reading and driving!)—pull over, stop, take off your shoes and socks, get out and stand up.

In the library or a bookstore? People are giving you funny looks as you remove your socks, aren't they? Better go home before you get arrested.

All set? Read the rest of this paragraph, then shut your eyes and follow the instructions. And here they are: Stand normally, relax; let your feet, shoulders and head go where they want to go (and do go when someone isn't barking out orders). Keep your feet in place, inhale and exhale a couple of times. Take your time. Notice how your weight is distributed. One leg will be working harder than the other. Is it the right leg? Left? Feel where the weight settles in the feet— heels? Inside edge, outside edge, toward the toes? It's likely to be in a different spot in each foot. Let two or three minutes go by. Breathe.

Now, open your eyes. Read some more. Did you notice what was going through your mind when you were analyzing the weight distribution? Was there a jumble of ideas, images, and sensations? A little of this and that? Quick arrhythmic bursts of activity? A sensory jigsaw puzzle with a bunch of missing pieces? At the end of this paragraph, close your eyes again and pay attention to your mental traffic. Give it a minute and reopen your eyes.

Now I'd like you to balance your weight distribution evenly. Read this paragraph and close your eyes again. Edge both feet around until they're roughly parallel, pointing straight ahead and about hips-width apart. Now, turn them inward a little, till they are slightly pigeon-toed. Easy does it. Carefully swing your torso, shoulders and head around until you can feel the weight move in your feet. Did you ever play flashlight tag as a kid? The beam of light moved like a disc, right? The weight will have the same characteristic; it will focus and slide here and there. Nudge the discs into the balls of your feet. Bob a little at the knees, tweak your hips. Some people will really have to crank themselves around. It may feel strange, precarious. Believe me, though, when the weight rests over the balls of the feet, your posture is in a balanced position. (The contortions and muscular effort to hold you there are necessary because your musculoskeletal structure is fighting to pop out of the temporary alignment that I've put you in.)

When you get the weight centered, notice how it feels, notice what your mind is doing. Go ahead, try it.

When we have our clients perform the same exercise in one of our Egoscue Method clinics, most of them say that in the first unbalanced position their minds are whirling, jumpy and chaotic. They feel troubled, uncertain, uneasy. Balanced, however, is a different story. The mind calms down. It loses the jittery quality. There's more steadiness and clarity.

We are just a small step away from entering the end zone unique to all literary ventures. It is the point where the author and his readers part company after spending, in our case, 195 pages together being buffeted by words and ideas. It is nearly impossible to resist over-explaining. Just one more metaphor, another example, an eye-catching statistic begs to be sent into the game in the last few minutes of play. Yet even the most stubbornly loquacious know it is too late. By now, you get it or you don't. The little girl who greeted us on the front cover of **LET'S LIGHTEN UP** gets it. She feels good catching the rain, living totally in the moment. Let her image into your heart.

Source Notes

An Informal Introduction

Pg v–Ralph Waldo Emerson. This epigram appears on many Internet Web sites, including Laura Moncur's *Motivational Quotations*, where I originally encountered it: quotation #3155. Originally published in Emerson's first collection of essays in 1841. Emerson, one of the founding fathers of American letters, edited the *Dial* magazine; he was a poet, essayist, and philosopher. You can find the entire essay at http://www.emersoncentral.com/selfreliance.htm.

Pg vii–"... photos snapped by Apollo...." The rhetorical trope "Spaceship Earth" was first suggested in a July 9, 1965 speech to the United Nations by Adlai E. Stevenson, the U.S. envoy to the world body: "We travel together, passengers on a little space ship, dependent on its vulnerable reserves of air and soil." Popular books by British economist Barbara Ward and technologist Buckminster Fuller elaborated on the spaceship analogy, and the term was linked with dramatic photographs of planet Earth recorded by Apollo astronauts and made into posters and T-shirts. (See Chris C. Park, *The Environment*: *Principles and Applications;* Routledge, 2001, page 99, and *The World Almanac,* 1965).

Media guru and iconoclast Marshall McLuhan reputedly said "There are no passengers on spaceship earth. We are all crew." From www.IWise.com, Wisdom on Demand, a Web site.

Thomas J. Friedman, *The World Is Flat: A Brief History of the Twenty-First Century*; Picador, 2007. Friedman is a New York Times op-ed columnist.

Pg viii–The author of "Pain is inevitable, suffering is optional." was an anonymous Buddhist priest. The adage is widely quoted. See Thich Nhat Hanh, *The Heart of the Buddha's Teachings*: *Transforming Suffering into Peace, Joy, and Liberation*: Broadway Books, page 105.

Four previous Egoscue works of nonfiction co-authored with Roger Gittines are in print: *Pain Free for Women, Pain Free at Your PC, Pain Free* and *The Egoscue Method of Health through Motion.*

Pg ix–"… a million years' worth…." I'm a contrarian on the subject of when the first genuine human walked the earth. The missing link is missing because we have, I believe, been searching in the wrong time periods. The basic human package that we know as Homo sapiens has been around for longer than a million years, not 200,000, the estimate based on an exasperatingly incomplete fossil record (due to natural causes, not conspiracies). My hypothesis is that our direct, earliest ancestors at first lived on the margins with various semi-compatible primate species and humanoid precursor-species like Neanderthal that were episodically tolerant and hostile to the odd, seemingly non-threatening creatures. Skittish, rare, relatively small in size and number, Homo sapiens may have been captured and kept as pets or mascots valued somewhat for their intelligence, ability to fashion tools and trinkets, and a vocal gift that could soothe and arouse emotions (known today as singing). They had no cultural footprint and did not formally bury their dead for many thousands of years. Their fossil remains were scattered, fragile and are mistaken for those of smallish extinct primates and mammals. There are great chunks of time–millions of years–that have yet to yield a single fossil although we are certain that living species existed. Read Bill Bryson's book *A Short History of Nearly Everything* for a marvelously succinct and entertaining treatment of this subject.

"... 60 trillion...." No one knows for sure how many cells are packed into the human body. Undoubtedly the total varies somewhat from individual to individual. As a general estimate, 60 trillion or more is a guess often cited by many credible sources (among them Bill Bryson). I've seen estimates of as high as 200 trillion.

"... knowing better...." Awareness, memory, and choice are recurring themes of this book. Modern life has dimmed awareness with an ego-driven compulsion to live outside the present in either constant review of the past or in previews of the future.

Chapter 1, Good Cause

Pg 1–Epigram: Joseph Campbell, Bill Moyers, and Betty Sue Flowers (editor); see chapter one, "Myth and the Modern World," in *The Power of Myth;* Anchor, 1991. The book was based on a series of PBS interviews of Campbell conducted by Moyers.

Pg 9–"... pivot-point...." Esther M. Sternberg, M.D, *The Balance Within: The Science Connecting Health and Emotions;* W.H. Freeman, 2008. Sternberg does a fine job of pulling together recent research on the mind-body-heath connection, though she does not address the musculoskeletal system issues that I regard as being of central importance.

Pg 10–"Extinction is the rule...." Bill Bryson, *A Short History of Almost Everything;* Broadway Books, 2003. Here is the first of many science gleanings from the marvelously lucid and concise Bryson (the second if you count "60 trillion cells;" see above).

Pg 10–"... ATP...." Stedman's Medical Dictionary, 25th Anniversary Edition; Stedmans, 1990.

"... brain of the cell...." Bruce H. Lipton, *The Biology of Belief;* Hay House, page 101.

"... two-way negotiations...." Colin Tudge, *The Tree: A Natural History of What Trees Are, How They Live, and Why They Matter;* Crown, page 82. His *The Time Before History* is also excellent and was an important source for *Pain Free*.

Pg 11–"Emotional intelligence...." Daniel Goleman, *Emotional Intelligence;* Bantam, 1995. A timely, classic treatment on the subject of emotions and how they influence success in life.

Pg 13–"There is no requirement...." Susan Blackmore, *Consciousness: A Very Short Introduction.* Oxford University Press, 2005.

Chapter 3, Your Fuel Gauge

Pg 36–"*Der Fliegende Holländer* (The Flying Dutchman)." Kobbe's Complete Opera Book edited and revised by the Earl of Harewood; Putnam and Company, 1976.

Pg 38–"... chowder...." Bryson again at his best.

Pg. 47–"... medicine a good name...." W. Grant Thompson, *The Placebo Effect and Health: Combining Science & Compassionate Care*; Prometheus Books, 2005.

Chapter 6, Balance of Forces

Pg 80–"The feel of things rather than the think of things" or words to that effect were either said by Stanley Kubrick, or offered as an observation about him. The exact source cannot be nailed down. But I believe Kubrick deserves the credit.

Chapter 8, Storytellers

Pg 89—"Man of twists and turns...." Homer, *The Odyssey*. Translated by Robert Fagles; Viking, page 77.

Pg 90—"Gilgamesh" Translated from the Sin-Leqi-Unninni Version by John Gardner and John Maier; Knopf, page 6. One of the keys to understanding humankind's fate is Enkidu's realization (Odysseus's too) that nothing is permanent, and yet that is not cause for despair. Why then act at all? Gardner and Maier wonder and offer this: "because action is life."

—"Who's there?" William Shakespeare, *Hamlet*, Act 1, Scene 1.

Chapter 12, Making the Worst of It

Pg 144—"Stress & Your Heart" by Anne Underwood. Newsweek, Oct. 3, 2005, page 52.

Pg 145—"Emotion Rules the Brain's Decisions" By Dan Vergano, updated 8/6/2006, USA TODAY on line.

Pg 153, footnote—"Placebos Are Getting More Effective. Drug Makers Are Desperate to Know Why" by Steve Silberman; Wired Magazine, page 144.

Chapter 13, Unstick This

Pg 169—"Spirit ...." Science meets science courtesy of Bruce Lipton.

Pg 177—"The simple act of appreciation...." Deepak Chopra, *Quantum Healing: Exploring the Frontiers of Mind/Body Medicine*; Bantam, 1990.

Index

About the Authors

Pete Egoscue, a postural and exercise therapist since 1978 (what he describes as being a "posture guy"), developed the world's leading non-medical treatment program for relieving chronic pain associated with accidents, workplace and sports injuries, aging and other serious conditions that undermine the health of millions of people. To meet the heavy demand, there are twenty-four Egoscue Method clinics in the United States, Europe and Asia. The unique national and international network is reinforced by hundreds of independent physicians, trainers, chiropractors and other recognized specialists with extensive experience and mandatory certification in Pete's signature methodology that greatly expands treatment options. The Egoscue Research Foundation underwrites and conducts cutting-edge musculoskeletal system research. "The Patch™," a nonprofit educational foundation, strives to improve the health and fitness of children. Pete Egoscue is also co-author with Roger Gittines of *Pain Free at Your PC, Pain Free Women, Pain Free: A Revolutionary Method for Stopping Chronic Pain* and *The Egoscue Method of Health through Motion.*

E-mail him at: Pete@Egoscue.com, or visit his Web site: www.Egoscue.com.

Also on Twitter, YouTube, Facebook and on Internet radio, Pain Free Radio.

Roger Gittines is a journalist and writer based in Washington, DC. His e-mail address is: rgittines@aol.com.

Also by Pete Egoscue with Roger Gittines

**Pain Free: A Revolutionary Method for Stopping
Chronic Pain**

"Shows how we can break the circuit of pain and
naturally heal one of the most significant disabilities of
our time."

Deepak Chopra

**Pain Free for Women: The Revolutionary Method for
Ending Chronic Pain**

"Thanks to Pete Egoscue, I've been pain free for ten
years...."

Carol LeBeau, Health reporter, KGTV, San Diego

**Pain Free at Your PC: Using a Computer Doesn't Have
to Hurt**

"Straight talk ... brilliant insights ... an important
book...."

James V. Kimsey, founding CEO of AOL

**The Egoscue Method of Health through Motion:
A Revolutionary Program that Let's You Rediscover the
Body's Power to Protect and Rejuvenate Itself**

"Read this book. But more importantly, use it."

Tony Robbins